# The complete
# FIBROMYALGIA
## Cookbook

By:

Maria Lancasters

# TABLE OF CONTENTS

**INTRODUCTION** ............................................................... 8

**Fibromyalgia Recipes** .................................................. 11

    1  The Best Avocado Toast ................................... 11

    2 Glazed sesame salmon ...................................... 13

    3 Greek-Style Chicken Salad ............................... 15

    4 Lemon Pepper Zucchini .................................... 17

    5 Apple Cherry Baked Oatmeal .......................... 18

    6  Roasted Red Pepper and Tomato Soup ....... 20

    7 Minty Pea Salad .................................................. 22

    8  Chana Aloo Masala (Chickpea and Potato Masala) ........................................................................ 24

    9 Cucumber Tomato and Onion Salad ............. 27

    10 Sweet Chili Stir Fried Tofu Bowls ................. 29

    11 Pan Fried Sesame Tofu with Broccoli ......... 31

    12 Banana Coconut Baked Oatmeal ................. 34

    13 Plum Salad with Lemon Ginger Dressing . 36

    14 Spinach Mushroom French Bread Pizzas . 38

    15 Curried Red Lentil and Pumpkin Soup ...... 40

    16 Smoky Parmesan Roasted Cauliflower ..... 42

    17 Chili Lime Cantaloupe ..................................... 44

18 Apple Cabbage Slaw .................................... 46

19  One Pot Roasted Red Pepper Pasta ........... 48

20 Fluffy Garlic Herb Mashed Potatoes ........... 50

21 Vegetarian Sweet Potato Tacos with Lime Crema ................................................................. 52

22 Spanish Chickpeas and Rice ......................... 55

23  Homemade Crepes ....................................... 58

24 Dilly Vegetable Dip ........................................ 60

25 Sweet Potato Cornbread ............................... 61

26 Vegetarian Mustard Greens ......................... 64

27 Vegetable Enchilada Casserole .................... 66

28 Triple Berry Oatmeal Muffins ...................... 69

29 Cabbage and Cranberry Salad ..................... 72

30 Creamy Pesto Mac and Cheese with Spinach ............................................................................. 73

31 Banana Nut Breakfast Farro ........................ 75

32 Fresh Apple Pie Scones ................................. 77

33 Eggs Florentine Breakfast Pizza .................. 80

34 Oven Roasted Frozen Broccoli .................... 83

35 Easy Homemade Cornbread Recipe ........... 85

36 Poor Man's Burrito Bowls ............................. 87

37 Roasted Red Pepper Hummus Wraps ........ 89

38 Mediterranean Farro Salad with Spiced Chickpeas ............................................................ 91

39 Vegetarian Shepherd's Pie............................ 94

40 5 Minute Nacho Cheese Sauce..................... 97

41 Caramelized Banana and Peanut Butter Quesadilla ................................................................ 99

42 Easy Spinach Ricotta Pasta .......................... 101

43 Easy Hot and Sour Soup with Vegetables and Tofu ................................................................... 103

44 Spinach and Chickpea Rice Pilaf ................ 105

45 Homemade Naan Bread Recipe ................. 107

46 Pineapple Sriracha Breakfast Bowls........ 110

47 Chili Roasted Sweet Potatoes..................... 112

48 Creamy Spinach Artichoke Pizza............... 114

49 Smoky Tomato Soup ...................................... 117

50 Cheddar Grits Breakfast Bowls .................. 119

51 Garden Vegetable Quinoa Soup ................. 121

52 Savory Vegetarian Stuffing Recipe........... 124

53 Chili Garlic Tofu Bowls .................................. 127

54 Roasted Apple Cranberry Relish ............... 130

55 Creamy Mushroom Herb Pasta .................. 132

56 "Oatmeal Cookie" Baked Oatmeal.............. 135

57 Crispy Hash Browns ....................................... 137

58 Weeknight Enchiladas................................... 139

59 Tropical Yogurt Parfaits ............................... 142

60 Broiled Balsamic Vegetables with Lemon Parsley Rice..................144

61 Sesame Kale ..................148

62 Blueberry Buttermilk Coffee Cake............150

63 Broccoli Cheddar Stuffed Baked Potatoes ..................152

64 Chimichurri Sauce: Good on Anything and Everything ..................155

65 Kale Salad with Cajun Spiced Chickpeas and Buttermilk Dressing..................157

66 Slow Cooker Coconut Curry Lentils..........160

67 Veggie Packed Freezer Breakfast Sandwiches..................162

68 Homemade Pineapple Orange Julius.......164

69 No-Churn Mint Chocolate Chip Ice Cream ..................165

70 Ultimate Southwest Scrambled Eggs........167

71 Cheddar Grits Breakfast Bowls..................169

72 Chipotle Portobello Oven Fajitas..................171

73 Tomato Herb Rice with White Beans and Spinach ..................173

74 Pressure Cooker Split Pea Soup..................176

75 Southwest Spaghetti Squash Bowls..........178

76 Freezer Ready Mini Pizzas..................180

77 Purple Power Bowls.................................182

78 Creamy Lemon Dill Greek Pasta Salad ....184

79 Parsley Scallion Hummus Pasta.................187

80 Cumin Rice..................................................189

81 Strawberry Rosé Slush................................191

82 Marinated Lentil Salad...............................192

83 Warm Corn and Avocado Salad.................195

84 Pickled Red Onions ...................................197

85 Harissa Roasted Vegetables.......................199

86 Cheesy Scallion Stuffed Jalapeños.............201

87 Tomato Herb Rice with White Beans and Spinach .........................................................203

88 Smoky White Bean Shakshuka...................206

89 Broccoli Salad with Honey Yogurt Dressing ........................................................................208

90 Ultimate Portobello Mushroom Pizza .....210

91 Peanut Butter and Jelly Bars......................213

92 Simple Homemade Cranberry Sauce .......215

93 5 Ingredient Freezer Biscuits ....................217

94 Anne Byrn's 1917 Applesauce Cake.........219

95 Lemon Butter Green Beans .......................221

96 Mango Coconut Tofu Bowls ......................223

97 Maple Brown Butter Mashed Sweet Potatoes ........................................................................227

98 Savory Cabbage Pancakes (Okonomiyaki) ...............................................................229

99 Pasta with 5 Ingredient Butter Tomato Sauce..........................................................232

100 Lemon Berry Cobbler................................235

101 Zucchini and Orzo Salad with Chimichurri ...............................................................238

CONCLUSION ................................................240

# INTRODUCTION

If you suffer from fibromyalgia it is important that you follow a balanced fibromyalgia diet to optimize healing. Many people don't realize how much food actually affects their body and symptoms, and a change in diet can really help to relieve the pain and discomfort associated with fibromyalgia. In developing your diet plan there will be foods you need to eliminate from your diet, and others that you will want to eat in abundance for maximum results. Let's take a look at a typical fibromyalgia diet plan that you may wish to follow.

Your fibromyalgia diet should be balanced in healthy, nutritious foods. Focus your eating habits around whole foods such as seeds, whole grains, raw fruits and raw vegetables, lean meats, and nuts. Basically, you want to stick to natural and un-processed foods as much as possible. When the processed foods are consumed, your symptoms may increase because of the refined sugars and flours.

Fruits and vegetable are high in "phytochemicals," it has been found that these can help reduce pain in those suffering from fibromyalgia. So eat plenty of fruits and vegetables, as many as you want! You will also want to drink plenty of water, at least 8 glasses a day. Many people who suffer from fibromyalgia have also found juicing to help with healing, because it allows them to get larger amounts of fruits and veggies quickly. Overall, simply eating a well balanced diet can boast amazing healing results.

There are also foods that you will want to eliminate from your diet so your body can begin to heal. Almost everything on the list should really not be surprising, since most of these foods are not considered healthy for any diet. It is good to pay attention to any foods that you are personally affected by-- if you notice that something makes you sick, then don't eat it!

Start paying close attention to food labels and eliminate from your diet foods that contain sugar, caffeine, white flour, preservatives, artificial sweeteners and nitrates. You will also want to avoid red meat, processed foods, carbonated beverages, chocolate, alcohol, and dairy products high in fat. Some people who suffer from fibromyalgia may also have sensitivity to acidic foods. Therefore, you may want to try eliminating acidic foods to see if you notice a difference.

You have just learned how following a good fibromyalgia diet plan can lead to healing results. Many sufferers of fibromyalgia report amazing results when they eliminate foods that can trigger fibromyalgia symptoms and eat a well balanced whole food diet. If you follow this eating plan you will not only begin the healing process for fibromyalgia, but you will also be eating to fight other diseases like cancer and heart disease. This diet plan is one you may want your entire family to follow with you.

# FIBROMYALGIA RECIPES

## 1  THE BEST AVOCADO TOAST

Prep Time: 20 minutes
Total Time: 20 minutes
Servings: 4 slices

### Ingredients

- 4 slices thick whole grain bread (or gluten-free equivalent)
- 1 large ripe avocado
- 1/3 cup frozen shelled edamame
- 1 lime
- 1 scallion (sliced thinly)
- 1/2 cup raw fresh corn kernels (1 ear)
- 1/2 cup tomato (diced)
- 1/2 cup cilantro (chopped)
- 1/4 cup hemp seeds (optional)
- salt to taste
- crushed red pepper flakes (to taste)
- olive oil (for drizzling)

### Instructions

- Toast the bread.
- Soak the edamame in warm water in a small bowl.
- Cut the corn off the cob and measure out 1/2 cup (save remaining corn for another use).
- Mash the edamame in a small bowl and then mash in the avocado.
- Add the sliced scallions and corn to the avocado/edamame mixture.
- Add the juice from half of the lime along with a sprinkle of salt, mix, and taste. Add more lime juice or salt as needed.
- When the toast is done, rub a cut garlic clove over the surface of each piece of toast.
- Spread the avocado mixture evenly onto each piece of toast.
- Top each slice with a drizzle of olive oil, crushed red pepper flakes, hemp seeds, tomato, and cilantro. You can also add a sprinkle of salt and lime juice if you like.

### *Nutrition Info*

Calories: 280kcal, Protein: 10g, Fat: 16.89g, Sodium: 738mg, Sugar: 4g

# 2 GLAZED SESAME SALMON

Prep:10 mins
Cook:15 mins - 20 mins
Plus marinating
Servings 4

## *Ingredients*

- 2 tbsp chilli sauce (we used sriracha)
- 2 tbsp soy sauce
- 1 tbsp sesame oil
- 1 tbsp rice wine
- 1 garlic clove , crushed
- 2 tsp finely grated ginger
- 4 salmon fillets
- 1 tbsp sesame seeds
- boiled rice , to serve
- stir-fried vegetables , to serve

## *Instructions*

- Heat oven to 200C/180C fan/gas 6. In a shallow dish, mix together the chilli sauce, soy, sesame oil, rice wine, garlic and ginger. Lay the pieces of salmon in the marinade, skin-side up, and set aside for 15 mins.
- Put the marinated salmon on a baking tray, skin-side down, and spoon over a little of the leftover

marinade. Sprinkle with the sesame seeds and roast in the oven for 15 mins, or until done to your liking. Serve with steamed rice and stir-fried vegetables.

# 3 GREEK-STYLE CHICKEN SALAD

Hands-on Time 20 Mins
Total Time 25 Mins
Servings 1

## Ingredients

- Pita chips: 1 1/2 (6-inch) whole-wheat pitas, cut into 11 wedges Cooking spray
- 1/4 teaspoon ground cumin
- 1/4 teaspoon paprika
- 1/4 teaspoon dried oregano

Chicken salad:

- 2 tablespoons chopped red onion
- 1 tablespoon canola mayonnaise
- 1 tablespoon plain 2% reduced-fat Greek yogurt
- 1 teaspoon fresh lemon juice
- 1/8 teaspoon black pepper
- 2 ounces chopped skinless, boneless rotisserie chicken (about 1 cup)

Parsley salad:

- 3/4 cup chopped fresh flat-leaf parsley
- 1/3 cup cherry tomatoes, halved 1/2 cup chopped English cucumber

- 2 tablespoons chopped red onion
- 2 teaspoons fresh lemon juice
- 2 teaspoons olive oil

## *Instructions*

- Preheat oven to 400°.
- To prepare pita chips, arrange pita wedges on a baking sheet; coat with cooking spray. Combine cumin, paprika, and oregano in a small bowl; sprinkle over pita wedges. Bake at 400° for 10 minutes or until toasted. Reserve 5 pita chips for another use.
- To prepare chicken salad, combine 2 tablespoons chopped red onion and next 5 ingredients (through chicken) in a bowl.
- To prepare parsley salad, combine parsley and remaining ingredients in a bowl; top with 1/2 cup chicken salad and remaining 6 pita chips.

## *Nutrition Info*

Calories 394 Fat 17.2g Satfat 2.2g Monofat 10g Polyfat 3.2g Protein 25g Carbohydrate 38g Fiber 7g Cholesterol 51mg Iron 5mg Sodium 588mg Calcium 117mg

# 4 LEMON PEPPER ZUCCHINI

Prep Time: 5 mins
Cook Time: 20 mins
Total Time: 25 mins
Servings: 4

## *Ingredients*

- 1 to 1.5 lbs. zucchini
- 1 Tbsp olive oil
- 1/2 Tbsp (or to taste) Lemon Pepper Seasoning

## *Instructions*

- Rinse the zucchini, remove the ends, then cut into 1/4 to 1/2 inch thick medallions. Place the medallions in a bowl, drizzle with olive oil, and sprinkle with lemon pepper. Toss the zucchini until evenly coated in oil and seasoning.
- Preheat the grill (for a George Foreman, I turn it on for about 5 minutes to preheat). Cook the medallions until they are tender and lightly browned on each side (about 3-4 minutes per side). Serve warm.

# 5 APPLE CHERRY BAKED OATMEAL

Prep Time: 10 mins
Cook Time: 45 mins
Total Time: 55 mins
Servings: 6

## *Ingredients*

- 1/2 tsp almond extract
- 1/4 tsp cinnamon
- 1/4 tsp salt
- 1 cup frozen pitted sweet cherries
- 1 1/2 cups unsweetened applesauce
- 2 large eggs
- 1/2 tsp vanilla extract
- 3/4 tsp baking powder
- 1 cup milk
- 2 cups uncooked old fashioned rolled oats

## *Instructions*

- Take the cherries out of the freezer and allow them to thaw. Preheat the oven to 375 degrees.
- In a large bowl, whisk together the apple sauce, eggs, vanilla and almond extracts, cinnamon, salt, and baking powder. Once combined, add the milk and whisk until smooth.

- Roughly chop the cherries and add them to the bowl of liquid ingredients, along with the rolled oats. Stir with a spoon until combined.
- Lightly coat an 8"x8" or 9"x9" baking dish with non-stick spray. Pour the oat mixture into the dish and then bake for 40-45 minutes, or until golden brown on top and no longer tacky in the center. Divide into six portions and serve warm.

## *Nutrition Info*

Calories: 189.62kcal, Carbohydrates: 30.05g, Protein: 7.08g, Fat: 4.85g, Sodium: 185.37mg, Fiber: 3.82g

# 6 ROASTED RED PEPPER AND TOMATO SOUP

Prep Time: 10 mins
Cook Time: 15 mins
Total Time: 25 mins
Servings: (1.5 cups each)

## *Ingredients*

- 2 Tbsp butter
- 1 yellow onion
- 4 cloves garlic
- 2 Tbsp all-purpose flour
- 2 15oz. cans crushed tomatoes
- 1 12oz. jar roasted red peppers
- 2 cups vegetable broth*
- 1/4 tsp dried basil
- 1/8 tsp dried thyme
- Freshly cracked black Pepper
- 1 cup whole milk (optional)

## *Instructions*

- Dice the onion and mince the garlic. Add the onion, garlic, and butter to a large soup pot. Sauté over a medium flame until the onions are soft and transparent (about 5 minutes).
- Add the flour to the pot and continue to stir and cook for 1-2 minutes. The flour will form a paste

with the butter and onions and begin to coat the bottom of the pot. As soon as the flour that is stuck to the pot begins to turn slightly golden, remove it from the heat.
- Add the crushed tomatoes (with juices), roasted red peppers (without juices) and the flour paste from the soup pot to a food processor or blender. Blend until smooth, then return the contents to the soup pot.
- Add the vegetable broth, basil, thyme, and some freshly cracked pepper (10-15 cranks of a pepper mill) to the soup and stir to combine. Heat and stir over a medium flame until the soup begins to simmer. Use the spoon to help dissolve any flour stuck to the bottom of the pot as you stir.
- Once the soup begins to simmer, turn off the heat. Add the milk, if using, and stir to combine. Taste and add salt if needed (this will depend on the salt content of your broth).

### *Nutrition Info*

Calories: 240.8kcal, Carbohydrates: 34.48g, Protein: 6.6g, Fat: 7.85g, Sodium: 1020.35mg, Fiber: 4.3g

# 7 MINTY PEA SALAD

Prep Time: 20 mins
Total Time: 20 mins
Servings: (3/4 cup each)

## *Ingredients*

- 1 lb. frozen peas
- 1 fresh lemon
- 1 small shallot, minced (about 2 Tbsp)
- 2 Tbsp olive oil
- 1/4 tsp salt
- Freshly cracked pepper
- 3-4 sprigs fresh mint

## *Instructions*

- Let the peas thaw in a colander to allow excess moisture to drain away. Rinsing briefly with cool water will expedite the thawing process.
- While the peas are thawing, prepare the lemon and shallot vinaigrette. Zest the lemon using a zester or a small holed cheese grater. Be sure to scrape off just the yellow zest and none of the bitter white pith. Set the zest aside, then squeeze about 2 tablespoons of the juice into a separate bowl.

- Peel the dry, papery skin from the shallot, then mince it finely. Add it to the bowl with the lemon juice, along with 2 Tbsp olive oil, 1/4 tsp salt, and some freshly cracked pepper (5-10 cranks of a pepper mill). Whisk the ingredients together until combined, then set aside.
- Rinse the mint to remove any dirt or debris. Pull the leaves from the stems and then slice into thin strips (or chop roughly).
- Add the thawed peas to a large bowl along with the vinaigrette, mint, and a hefty pinch of the lemon zest. Stir to combine, then taste and add more zest if desired. Serve immediately, or refrigerate to allow the flavors to blend.

### *Nutrition Info*

Calories: 117kcal, Carbohydrates: 11.03g, Protein: 3.53g, Fat: 7.18g, Sodium: 213.4mg, Fiber: 4.33g

# 8 CHANA ALOO MASALA (CHICKPEA AND POTATO MASALA)

Prep Time: 10 mins
Cook Time: 25 mins
Total Time: 35 mins
Servings: 4

## *Ingredients*

- 1 lb. russet potato
- 2 Tbsp olive oil
- 1 yellow onion
- 2 cloves garlic
- 2 Tbsp grated fresh ginger
- 1 Tbsp garam masala (or to taste)
- 1 28oz. can crushed tomatoes
- 2 Tbsp tomato paste
- 1/2 tsp salt (or to taste)
- 1 15oz. can chickpeas
- 1/4 bunch fresh cilantro (optional)
- 6 oz. plain yogurt (optional)
- 4 cups cooked rice (optional)

## *Instructions*

- Peel the potato and cut it into one-inch cubes. Place the cubes in a sauce pot, add enough water to cover the potatoes by one inch, and bring the

pot to a boil over high heat. Boil the potatoes for 5-7 minutes, or until they can easily be pierced with a fork. Drain the potatoes and set them aside.
- Dice the onion, mince the garlic, and peel and grate the ginger (use a small-holed cheese grater). Add the olive oil, onion, garlic, and ginger to a large deep skillet and sauté over medium heat until the onions are soft and transparent (3-5 minutes).
- Add the garam masala to the skillet and continue to sauté for about a minute more to toast the spices. It's okay if the spices begin to stick to the surface of the skillet slightly, but be sure not to let them burn.
- Add the crushed tomatoes and tomato paste to the skillet. Stir to dissolve the tomato paste into the crushed tomatoes and to dissolve the spices off the bottom of the skillet. Allow the sauce to heat through (about five minutes). Taste the sauce and add salt as needed (I added 1/2 tsp salt).
- Drain the chickpeas, then add them to the skillet along with the cooked potatoes. Stir everything to coat in the hot sauce, then heat through. Spoon the Chana Aloo Masala over cooked rice (or serve with naan), topped with chopped cilantro and a dollop of plain yogurt (regular or Greek style).

***Nutrition Info***

Calories: 636.4kcal, Carbohydrates: 111.68g, Protein: 21.3g, Fat: 12.73g, Sodium: 1362.1mg, Fiber: 15.23g

# 9 CUCUMBER TOMATO AND ONION SALAD

Prep Time: 20 mins
Total Time: 20 mins
Servings: to 6 servings

## Ingredients

DRESSING

- 1/4 cup olive oil
- 2 Tbsp red wine vinegar
- 1 tsp dried oregano
- 1/2 tsp salt
- Freshly cracked pepper

SALAD

- 4 Roma tomatoes (or two medium tomatoes)
- 1 cucumber
- 1/2 red onion

## Instructions

- Whisk together the olive oil, red wine vinegar, oregano, salt, and some freshly cracked pepper in a bowl, or combine them in a jar and shake until mixed. Set the dressing aside to allow the flavors to blend.

- Thinly slice* the tomato, cucumber, and red onion. Place them in a large bowl.
- Pour the dressing over the sliced vegetables and toss to coat. Serve immediately, or refrigerate until ready to eat. The onions will become more mild as they marinate in the dressing.

**Nutrition Info**

Calories: 142.65kcal, Carbohydrates: 4.7g, Protein: 1g, Fat: 13.73g, Sodium: 360.48mg, Fiber: 1.48g

# 10 SWEET CHILI STIR FRIED TOFU BOWLS

Prep Time: 45 mins
Cook Time: 10 mins
Total Time: 55 mins
Servings: 4

## *Ingredients*

- 14 oz. extra firm tofu
- 1 pinch salt
- 2 Tbsp cornstarch
- 2 Tbsp cooking oil*
- 1 avocado
- 1 bell pepper (any color)
- 2-3 green onions
- 1 handful fresh cilantro (optional
- 1/2 cup sweet chili sauce
- 2 tsp sesame seeds (optional)
- 4 cups cooked rice

## *Instructions*

- Remove the tofu from the liquid in the package, wrap it in a clean, lint-free dishcloth or a few paper towels, and press it between two plates with a weight on top for 30 minutes (see detailed step by step photos and instructions here). Once the excess moisture has been

pressed out, cut the tofu into 3/4 to 1-inch cubes.
- Season the tofu cubes with a pinch of salt. Sprinkle a tablespoon of cornstarch over top and then toss to coat. Repeat with the second tablespoon of cornstarch.
- Heat the oil in a large skillet over medium flame. Once the skillet and oil are hot, add the tofu cubes and fry until golden brown and crispy on all sides. Place the fried tofu in a large bowl.
- Dice the red bell pepper and thinly slice the green onions. Pull the cilantro leaves from the stems and give them a rough chop. Slice the avocado.
- Add the diced bell pepper to the bowl with the fried tofu. Pour 1/3 to 1/2 cup sweet chili sauce over top, then stir until the bell pepper and tofu are coated in the sauce.
- To build the bowls, start with one cup cooked rice, then add 1/4 of the tofu and bell pepper mixture. Add a few slices of avocado to the side of the bowl, then sprinkle the sliced green onion, chopped cilantro, and sesame seeds over top. Enjoy!

### Nutrition Info

Calories: 550.6kcal, Carbohydrates: 75.68g, Protein: 16.05g, Fat: 20.2g, Sodium: 919.23mg, Fiber: 6.1g

# 11 PAN FRIED SESAME TOFU WITH BROCCOLI

Prep Time: 45 mins
Cook Time: 15 mins
Total Time: 1 hr
Servings: 3

## *Ingredients*

SAUCE

- 1/4 cup soy sauce
- 2 Tbsp water
- 1 Tbsp toasted sesame oil
- 2 Tbsp brown sugar
- 2 Tbsp rice vinegar
- 1 Tbsp grated fresh ginger
- 2 cloves garlic, minced
- 2 Tbsp sesame seeds
- 1 Tbsp cornstarch

STIR FRY

- 14 oz block extra-firm tofu
- Pinch of salt
- 2 Tbsp cornstarch
- 2 Tbsp neutral oil (vegetable, canola, peanut)
- 1/2 lb frozen broccoli florets
- 3-4 green onions, sliced

- 4 cups cooked rice

**Instructions**

- Place a few folded paper towels or a clean, lint-free dish cloth on a large plate. Remove the tofu from the package and place it on the towels. Place more towels on top, cover with a second plate, and then weigh the top plate down with a few canned goods or a pot filled with water. Press the tofu for at least 30 minutes to extract excess water (refrigerate if pressing for longer).
- While the tofu is pressing, prepare the sauce so that the flavors have time to blend. In a small bowl combine the soy sauce, water, sesame oil, brown sugar, rice vinegar, grated ginger, minced garlic, sesame seeds, and cornstarch. Stir until the brown sugar and cornstarch are dissolved, then set the sauce aside.
- Cut the pressed tofu into 1-inch cubes, then season with a pinch of salt. Sprinkle 1 Tbsp cornstarch over the cubes, then toss to coat. Repeat with the second tablespoon of cornstarch, or until the tofu cubes have a nice even coating of cornstarch.
- Heat a large skillet over medium flame. Once hot, add 2 Tbsp oil and tilt the skillet until the bottom is coated in a thick layer of oil. Add the dusted tofu cubes and let cook until golden

brown on the bottom. Use a spatula to turn the cubes to an uncooked side, and cook until golden brown again. Continue this process until brown and crispy on all sides, then remove the crispy tofu to a clean plate.
- Add the frozen broccoli to the hot skillet and briefly stir fry until slightly browned on the edges. Don't worry if it's not thawed through yet, it will warm through after adding the sauce. Lower the heat to medium-low.
- Give the bowl of sauce a good stir, then pour it into the skillet with the broccoli. Stir and cook until the sauce begins to bubble and thicken (this should happen very quickly). Once thickened, turn off the heat and stir in the cooked tofu cubes.
- Serve the tofu and broccoli over a bed of cooked rice, topped with sliced green onions.

### *Nutrition Info*

Calories: 647.07kcal, Carbohydrates: 85.93g, Protein: 24.4g, Fat: 28.13g, Sodium: 1881.13mg, Fiber: 6.03g

## 12 BANANA COCONUT BAKED OATMEAL

Prep Time: 10 mins
Cook Time: 45 mins
Total Time: 55 mins
Servings: 6

### *Ingredients*

- 1.5 cups mashed ripe bananas
- 1 large egg
- 1/4 cup brown sugar
- 1/2 tsp vanilla
- 1/2 tsp nutmeg
- 1 tsp baking powder
- 1/2 tsp salt
- 1/3 cup unsweetened shredded coconut
- 1 13.5oz. can coconut milk
- 3 cups old-fashioned rolled oats

### *Instructions*

- Preheat the oven to 375ºF. Coat the inside of a 2-3 quart casserole dish with non-stick spray.
- In a large bowl, whisk together the mashed bananas, egg, brown sugar, vanilla, nutmeg, baking powder, salt, and shredded coconut until evenly combined. Add the coconut milk and

whisk until smooth again. Add the rolled oats and stir with a spoon until combined.
- Pour the oat mixture into the prepared casserole dish and bake, uncovered, for 45 minutes. Serve warm or refrigerate until ready to eat. Pairs well with cold milk poured over top.

### *Nutrition Info*

Calories: 320.4kcal, Carbohydrates: 53.05g, Protein: 7.28g, Fat: 9.52g, Sodium: 286.47mg, Fiber: 6.4g

# 13 PLUM SALAD WITH LEMON GINGER DRESSING

Prep Time: 20 mins
Total Time: 20 mins
Servings: 3 (1 cup each)

## *Ingredients*

- 1 tsp fresh grated ginger
- 2 Tbsp fresh lemon juice
- 3 Tbsp canola (or other light oil)
- 1 Tbsp honey
- 1/4 tsp salt
- Freshly cracked pepper
- 2 plums (about 1/2 lb. total)
- 1 bunch fresh parsley
- 1/4 cup sliced almonds
- 2 cups cooked bulgur, quinoa, couscous, or rice (chilled)

## *Instructions*

- Grate about one tsp of fresh ginger into a jar or small bowl. Add the lemon juice, salad oil, honey, salt, and some freshly cracked pepper. Shake the jar (or whisk) until the ingredients are combined. Let the dressing sit while you prepare the rest of the salad.

- Rinse the parsley well to remove any dirt or debris. Shake off as much water as possible. Pull the leaves from the stems and then give them a rough chop. Place the chopped parsley in a bowl.
- Thinly slice the plums and remove the sections from the pit. Add the plum slices and sliced almonds to the bowl with the parsley. Give the dressing a quick stir, then add it to the salad (start with half and add more as needed). Toss the salad until everything is coated in the dressing, then serve.

### *Nutrition Info*

Calories: 366.8kcal, Carbohydrates: 45.17g, Protein: 5.67g, Fat: 19.6g, Sodium: 542.6mg, Fiber: 3g

# 14 SPINACH MUSHROOM FRENCH BREAD PIZZAS

Prep Time: 10 mins
Cook Time: 20 mins
Total Time: 30 mins
Servings: 4

## *Ingredients*

- 3 Tbsp olive oil, divided
- 2 cloves garlic, minced
- 8 oz. button mushrooms
- 8 oz. frozen spinach
- salt & pepper to taste
- 1 16-inch loaf French bread
- 4 slices Swiss cheese

## *Instructions*

- Wipe the mushrooms clean, then slice thinly. Add 1 tablespoon of olive oil to a large skillet along with the minced garlic. Sauté the garlic over medium heat for one minute or just until fragrant. Add the sliced mushrooms and sauté for 3-5 minutes more, or until they are limp and dark brown (add a pinch of salt to help them release their moisture if needed).

- Add the frozen spinach to the skillet and continue to sauté until it is heated through. Season the mushrooms and spinach with salt and freshly cracked pepper to taste (I used about 1/4 tsp salt and 10 cranks of a pepper mill.
- Adjust your oven rack so that the top of the French bread will be 5-6 inches from the broiler unit. Preheat the broiler on high for a few minutes. While it's heating, cut the loaf of French bread into two 8 inch sections, then slice each piece in half lengthwise to open like a sandwich.
- Line a baking sheet with foil. Place the pieces of French bread on the baking sheet open side up. Brush the remaining 2 tablespoons of olive oil over the open surface of the bread. Place the bread under the broiler for about 3 minutes, or just until it is golden brown.
- Top each piece of bread with 1/4 of the spinach and mushroom mixture, and one piece of swiss. Return the topped bread to the oven and broil for 1-2 minutes, or just until the cheese is hot and bubbly. Watch them closely to prevent burning. Serve hot.

### *Nutrition Info*

Calories: 516.45kcal, Carbohydrates: 63.48g, Protein: 21.4g, Fat: 20.73g, Sodium: 1073.18mg, Fiber: 4.7g

## 15 CURRIED RED LENTIL AND PUMPKIN SOUP

Prep Time: 5 mins
Cook Time: 25 mins
Total Time: 30 mins
Servings: 4 (1.33 cups each)

### *Ingredients*

- 1 Tbsp olive oil
- 1 yellow onion
- 2 cloves garlic
- 1 Tbsp grated fresh ginger
- 1 15oz. can pumpkin purée
- 1 cup dry red lentils
- 6 cups vegetable broth
- 1 Tbsp curry powder (or to taste)

### *Instructions*

- Dice the onion, mince the garlic, and grate the ginger (use a small hole cheese grater). Sauté the onion, garlic, and ginger in a large pot with the olive oil over medium heat until the onions are soft and transparent.
- Add the pumpkin purée, red lentils, broth, and curry powder. Stir to combine.
- Place a lid on the pot, turn the heat up to medium-high, and allow it to come to a boil.

Once it reaches a boil, turn the heat down and simmer on low for 20 minutes, stirring occasionally. After 20 minutes the lentils should be soft and the soup slightly thickened.
- Taste to adjust the curry powder or salt as needed, then serve.

### *Nutrition Info*

Calories: 173.92kcal, Carbohydrates: 29.37g, Protein: 9.92g, Fat: 3.22g, Sodium: 863.92mg, Fiber: 4.85g

# 16 SMOKY PARMESAN ROASTED CAULIFLOWER

Prep Time: 15 mins
Cook Time: 45 mins
Total Time: 1 hr
Servings: 4 to 6 servings

## Ingredients

- 1 Tbsp smoked paprika
- 1/2 tsp dried oregano
- 1/4 tsp garlic powder
- 1/4 tsp salt
- Freshly cracked pepper
- 1/4 cup grated Parmesan
- 1 1/2 Tbsp olive oil
- 1 head cauliflower

## Instructions

- Preheat the oven to 400ºF. Prepare a baking sheet by covering it with foil and misting lightly with non-stick spray.
- In a small bowl, combine the smoked paprika, oregano, garlic powder, salt, freshly cracked pepper (10-15 cranks of a pepper mill), and grated Parmesan.

- Remove the leaves from the cauliflower, then cut into small florets. Place the florets in a large bowl and drizzle with olive oil. Toss the florets until they are evenly coated in oil. Add about 3/4 of the Parmesan spice mixture to the bowl and toss the florets until coated again.
- Spread the florets out over the surface of the baking sheet, making sure they are in a single layer. Add any Parmesan and spices left in the bottom of the bowl to the top of the florets, then sprinkle the remaining, unused portion of the Parmesan spice mix over top.
- Roast the cauliflower in the fully preheated oven for 40-45 minutes, or until the edges are browned and the cauliflower is tender. The parmesan will melt slightly and become crispy. Serve hot out of the oven.

### *Nutrition Info*

Calories: 107.75kcal, Carbohydrates: 9.1g, Protein: 4.48g, Fat: 7.1g, Sodium: 342.15mg, Fiber: 3.6g

# 17 CHILI LIME CANTALOUPE

Prep Time: 20 mins
Total Time: 20 mins
Servings: 4

## Ingredients

- 1/2 medium cantaloupe
- 1.5-2 Tbsp fresh lime juice (about 1/2 lime)
- 1/2 Tbsp honey
- 1/8 tsp salt
- 1/8 tsp crushed red pepper

## Instructions

- Cut the cantaloupe in half and scrape out the seeds with a spoon. Reserve half of the cantaloupe for breakfast or other meals. Take the remaining half and cut it into quarters. Using a sharp knife, carefully run the knife between the flesh and the rind. Once the rind is removed, slice the melon into thin pieces.
- In a small bowl, combine the juice of half a lime (about 1.5-2 Tbsp), honey, salt, and crushed red pepper. Stir until the honey is dissolved.
- Pour the dressing over the sliced cantaloupe and toss to coat the melon in the dressing. Serve

immediately, or chill until ready to eat. Give the melon a brief stir before serving.

### *Nutrition Info*

Calories: 33.45kcal, Carbohydrates: 8.48g, Protein: 0.6g, Fat: 0.13g, Sodium: 85.03mg, Fiber: 0.68g

# 18 APPLE CABBAGE SLAW

Prep Time: 20 mins
Total Time: 20 mins
Servings: (1 cup each)

## *Ingredients*

- 1/3 cup mayonnaise
- 1/3 cup Greek style plain yogurt
- 1 Tbsp apple cider vinegar
- 1/2 Tbsp honey
- 1/2 tsp salt
- 1 small head purple cabbage (about 1.5 lbs.)
- 1 carrot
- 1 Granny Smith apple
- 1/3 cup raisins

## *Instructions*

- Prepare the dressing by stirring together the mayonnaise, Greek yogurt, apple cider vinegar, honey, and salt.
- Remove the core from the cabbage, then shred the leaves into very thin strips. Peel the carrot, then shred it using a large holed cheese grater. Wash the apple well, slice it in half, then remove the core with a melon baller or sharp spoon. Use the cheese grater to shred the apple. Press the

shredded apple between a couple pieces of paper towel to absorb the excess juice.
- Place the shredded cabbage, carrot, apple, and raisins in a large bowl. Add the dressing over top, then stir until everything is evenly coated in dressing. Serve immediately.

### *Nutrition Info*

Calories: 218.42kcal, Carbohydrates: 25.91g, Protein: 3.62g, Fat: 12.86g, Sodium: 363.88mg, Fiber: 4.02g

# 19 ONE POT ROASTED RED PEPPER PASTA

Prep Time: 10 mins
Cook Time: 20 mins
Total Time: 30 mins
Servings: 6 (1 1/3 cup each)

## *Ingredients*

- 5 cups vegetable broth
- 1 lb. Fettuccine
- 1 small Vidalia onion
- 4 cloves garlic
- 1 12oz. jar roasted red peppers
- 1 15oz. can fire roasted diced tomatoes
- 1/2 Tbsp dried basil
- 1/4 tsp crushed red pepper (optional)
- Freshly cracked black pepper
- 4 oz. cream cheese (optional)

## *Instructions*

- Thinly slice the onion and mince the garlic. Remove the red peppers from the liquid in the jar and then slice them into thin strips.
- In a large pot, combine the broth, onion, garlic, red pepper slices, diced tomatoes (with juice), basil, crushed red pepper, and some freshly cracked black pepper (10-15 cranks of a pepper

mill). Stir these ingredients to combine. Break the fettuccine in half, then add it to the pot, attempting to submerge the pieces as much as possible.
- Place a lid on the pot and turn the heat up to high. As soon as the pot reaches a full boil, give it a quick stir to loosen any pieces that may have stuck to the bottom, return the lid, and turn the heat down to medium-low.
- Let the pot simmer on medium low for 10-12 minutes, stirring every couple of minutes to make sure nothing sticks to the bottom. Return the lid as quickly as possible after each stir. After ten minutes, test the pasta to see if it is al dente. Once the pasta is tender, remove it from the heat. (If the pasta becomes too dry before it is tender, simply add a small amount of water and continue to simmer.)
- Divide the cream cheese into tablespoon sized pieces, then add them to the pot. Stir the pasta until the cheese melts in and creates a smooth sauce (it will look lumpy at first, just keep stirring). Serve hot.

### *Nutrition Info*

Calories: 410.38kcal, Carbohydrates: 71.48g, Protein: 12.02g, Fat: 7.72g, Sodium: 1049.45mg, Fiber: 3.4g

## 20 FLUFFY GARLIC HERB MASHED POTATOES

Prep Time: 20 mins
Cook Time: 15 mins
Total Time: 35 mins
Servings: 1 cup each

### *Ingredients*

- 2.5 lbs. russet potatoes
- 1/2 tsp salt
- 4 Tbsp butter
- 1/2 cup whole milk

All-Purpose Garlic Herb Seasoning

- 1 tsp dried parsley
- 1/2 tsp dried oregano
- 1/2 tsp dried basil
- 1/4 tsp garlic powder
- 1/4 tsp onion powder
- 1/4 tsp salt
- freshly cracked pepper

### *Instructions*

- Peel and cut the russet potatoes into 1-inch cubes. Place the cubed potatoes in a colander and rinse well with cool water.

- Place the rinsed potatoes in a pot and add enough water to cover the potatoes by one inch. Season the water with 1/2 tsp salt. Cover the pot and bring it to a boil over high heat. Boil the potatoes until they are VERY tender, about 7-10 minutes.
- Drain the cooked potatoes in a colander, then rinse briefly with hot water.
- Add the butter, milk, and garlic herb seasoning o the pot used to boil the potatoes. Stir and heat over low until the butter has melted and the milk is hot.
- Once the milk is hot, add the potatoes back to the pot, turn off the heat and mash with a potato masher. Once the potatoes are mostly mashed, use a hand mixer to briefly whip the potatoes until they are light and fluffy. Taste the potatoes and add salt to taste, if needed, then serve.

**Nutrition Info**

Calories: 220.18kcal, Carbohydrates: 34.32g, Protein: 4.55g, Fat: 8g, Sodium: 405.58mg, Fiber: 2.77g

# 21 VEGETARIAN SWEET POTATO TACOS WITH LIME CREMA

Prep Time: 20 mins
Cook Time: 20 mins
Total Time: 40 mins
Servings: 4 (2 tacos per serving)

## *Ingredients*

Lime Crema

- 8 oz. sour cream
- 1 fresh lime
- 1/4 tsp salt
- 1 clove garlic

Tacos

- 1 Tbsp olive oil
- 2 cloves garlic
- 1.25 lbs. sweet potato
- 1 15oz. can black beans
- 1 tsp ground cumin
- Salt and Pepper to taste
- 2 green onions
- 1/4 bunch fresh cilantro (optional)
- 8 small (taco sized) tortillas

*Instructions*

- Prepare the crema first to allow the flavors time to blend. Mince one clove of garlic and use a zester or small holed cheese grater to scrape the thin layer of green zest from the lime. Add the minced garlic, 1 tsp of the zest, about 1 tsp of the lime juice, and 1/4 tsp salt to the sour cream. Stir the ingredients to combine then refrigerate until ready to use.
- Peel the sweet potatoes, then cut them into small cubes (about 1/4 to 1/2 inch square). Heat a large skillet over medium flame, then add the olive oil and two cloves of minced garlic. Sauté the garlic for about a minute or just until it becomes fragrant. Add the diced sweet potato and a couple tablespoons of water. Sauté the sweet potato until they become soft and just begin to fall apart. Add another couple tablespoons of water during cooking if the skillet becomes dry before the sweet potatoes are soft.
- Meanwhile, drain and rinse the can of black beans. Once the sweet potatoes are soft, add the black beans to the skillet. Season with the cumin, and salt and pepper to taste. Sauté just until the beans are heated through.
- Slice the green onions and pull the cilantro leaves from the stems. Roughly chop the cilantro. Stir the sliced green onions into the

skillet. Add the cilantro to the skillet if desired, or use it to top each taco.
- Prior to filling each tortilla, heat them in a dry skillet until slightly browned and crisp on each side, or carefully toast them over an open flame. Smear a small amount of the lime crema down the center of the tortilla, then top with a scoop of the sweet potato and black bean hash. Add fresh cilantro if desired.

### Nutrition Info

Calories: 655.85kcal, Carbohydrates: 88.6g, Protein: 18.75g, Fat: 26.48g, Sodium: 1502.13mg, Fiber: 17.4g

# 22 SPANISH CHICKPEAS AND RICE

Prep Time: 10 mins
Cook Time: 40 mins
Total Time: 50 mins
Servings: 4 (1.5 cups each)

## *Ingredients*

- 2 Tbsp olive oil
- 2 cloves garlic
- 1/2 Tbsp smoked paprika
- 1 tsp ground cumin
- 1/2 tsp dried oregano
- 1/4 tsp cayenne pepper
- Freshly cracked black pepper
- 1 yellow onion
- 1 cup uncooked long grain white rice
- 1 15oz. can diced tomatoes
- 1 15oz. can quartered artichoke hearts
- 1 19oz. can chickpeas
- 1.5 cups vegetable broth
- 1/2 tsp salt (or to taste)
- 1/4 bunch fresh parsley
- 1 fresh lemon

## *Instructions*

- Mince the garlic and add it to a large deep skillet along with the olive oil. Cook over medium-low heat for 1-2 minutes, or just until soft and fragrant. Add the smoked paprika, cumin, oregano, cayenne pepper, and some freshly cracked black pepper to the skillet. Stir and sauté the spices in the hot oil for one more minute.
- Dice the onion and add it to the skillet. Sauté the onion until it is soft and translucent (about 5 min). Add the rice and sauté for 2 minutes more.
- Drain the chickpeas and artichoke hearts, then add them to the skillet along with the can of diced tomatoes (with juices), vegetable broth, and a half teaspoon of salt. Roughly chop the parsley and add it to the skillet, reserving a small amount to sprinkle over the finished dish. Stir all the ingredients in the skillet until evenly combined.
- Place a lid on the skillet and turn the heat up to medium-high. Allow the skillet to come to a boil. Once it reaches a boil, turn the heat down to low and let simmer for 20 minutes. Make sure it's simmering the whole time and adjust the heat up slightly if necessary to keep it simmering.
- After simmering for 20 minutes, turn the heat off and let it rest for 5 minutes without removing the lid. Finally, remove the lid, fluff with a fork and top with the remaining chopped parsley. Cut

the lemon into wedges and squeeze the fresh juice over each bowl.

### *Nutrition Info*

Calories: 486.25kcal, Carbohydrates: 83.03g, Protein: 16.08g, Fat: 10.98g, Sodium: 1348.43mg, Fiber: 15.28g

# 23  HOMEMADE CREPES

Prep Time: 45 mins
Cook Time: 15 mins
Total Time: 1 hr
Servings: to 8 servings 8" crepes

## *Ingredients*

- 1/2 cup all-purpose flour
- 1/2 cup whole wheat flour
- 1/4 tsp salt
- 2 large eggs
- 3/4 cup milk
- 1/2 cup water
- 3 Tbsp butter, melted
- 1 tsp (or less) vegetable oil for cooking

## *Instructions*

- In a medium bowl, mix together the all-purpose flour, whole wheat flour, and salt. In a separate large bowl, whisk together the eggs, milk, and water until smooth. Add the flour mixture and melted butter to the whisked milk and eggs, then whisk again until no lumps remain.
- Cover the batter and refrigerate for 30 minutes or up to two days.

- When you're ready to make the crepes, lightly oil an 8" to 10" non-stick skillet. Pre-heat the skillet over medium flame. When the skillet is fully heated, scoop about 1/3 cup of the batter into the center of the skillet. Immediately lift the skillet and tilt it in a circular motion to allow the batter to run in a circular pattern and fill the bottom of the skillet. This is a quick motion and the batter should run and spread readily to a very thin layer on the surface of the skillet. If the batter is too thick to easily run and spread, whisk in a couple tablespoons of water and try again. If the skillet is too hot and the batter solidifies too fast, try lowering the heat a bit.
- Once the batter has spread over the surface of the skillet, return the skillet to the burner and cook until golden brown on the bottom. Flip and cook until golden brown on the second side. Remove the cooked crepe to a plate and start on the next one. Continue until all the batter has been used (6 to 8 8" crepes).

### *Nutrition Info*

Calories: 173.02kcal, Carbohydrates: 16.7g, Protein: 5.57g, Fat: 9.55g, Sodium: 179.78mg, Fiber: 1.35g

## 24 DILLY VEGETABLE DIP

Prep Time: 5 mins
Total Time: 5 mins
Servings: (2 Tbsp each)

### Ingredients

- 1/2 cup sour cream
- 1/4 tsp lemon pepper
- 1/4 tsp salt
- 1/16 tsp garlic powder
- 1 tsp chopped fresh dill

### Instructions

- In a small bowl, combine the sour cream, lemon pepper, salt, and garlic powder.
- Pull the wispy pieces of dill from the stems, then roughly chop. Stir the chopped dill into the sour cream. Taste and adjust the salt if needed.
- Serve immediately or refrigerate until ready to eat.

### Nutrition Info

Calories: 57.13kcal, Carbohydrates: 1.38g, Protein: 0.7g, Fat: 5.58g, Sodium: 191.6mg

## 25 SWEET POTATO CORNBREAD

Prep Time: 30 mins
Cook Time: 25 mins
Total Time: 55 mins
Servings: 8

### *Ingredients*

- 1 medium sweet potato (about 1 lb.)
- 1.5 cups yellow cornmeal
- 1 cup all-purpose flour
- 1/2 cup sugar
- 1 Tbsp baking powder
- 1 tsp salt
- 1/2 tsp cinnamon
- 1/2 tsp nutmeg
- 2 large eggs
- 1/2 cup sour cream
- 3/4 cup milk
- 2 Tbsp canola or vegetable oil
- 1/2 Tbsp canola or vegetable oil for the skillet

### *Instructions*

- Peel the sweet potato and cut it into one-inch cubes. Place the cubes in a pot, cover with water, and bring to a boil over high heat. Boil the potatoes until they're tender and fall apart with

pierced with a fork (about ten minutes). Drain the potatoes and set aside.
- Coat the inside of a 10-inch cast iron skillet with oil. Place it in the oven and begin to preheat the oven to 425 degrees.
- In a large bowl, stir together the cornmeal, flour, sugar, baking powder, salt, cinnamon, and nutmeg until well mixed.
- Mash the drained sweet potatoes until fairly smooth. Transfer 1.5 cups of the mashed potatoes to a large bowl. Add the sour cream, milk, and 2 Tbsp oil, and whisk until combined. Add the eggs and whisk until combined again.
- Pour the sweet potato mixture into the bowl with the dry ingredients. Stir the two together just until combined and no dry mix remains on the bottom of the bowl. It's okay if the mixture is a little lumpy, just be sure not to over mix.
- Carefully take the hot skillet out of the preheated oven and scoop the batter into it. Smooth the top out until it's even, then return it to the oven. Bake for 22-25 minutes, or until the center is puffed, the top is golden brown, and it's slightly cracked around the edges. Remove from the oven, cut into eight pieces, and serve. Preferably with butter.

**Nutrition Info**

Calories: 373.49kcal, Carbohydrates: 58.94g, Protein: 7.13g, Fat: 12.29g, Sodium: 570.19mg, Fiber: 3.15g

## 26 VEGETARIAN MUSTARD GREENS

Prep Time: 10 mins
Cook Time: 40 mins
Total Time: 50 mins
Servings: 6

### *Ingredients*

- 1 Tbsp olive oil
- 1 yellow onion
- 2 cloves garlic
- 2 cups vegetable broth*
- 1 lb. fresh mustard greens, stemmed and cut
- 1/2 Tbsp smoked paprika
- 1/2 Tbsp sugar
- Freshly cracked pepper
- 1 pinch crushed red pepper (optional)

### *Instructions*

- If your mustard greens did not come pre-cut and with stems removed, run a sharp knife down the center of each leaf to remove the woody stems. Cut the remaining leaves into 2-inch strips. Rinse the cut leaves well in a colander.
- Slice the onion thinly and mince the garlic. Sauté the onion and garlic in a large pot over medium heat with the olive oil until the onions are soft

(about 5 minutes). Add the vegetable broth and heat until steaming.
- Add the cut mustard greens, a couple handfuls at a time, stirring until wilted and there is room to add more to the pot. Once they're all mostly wilted, add the smoked paprika, sugar, some freshly cracked pepper, and a pinch of red pepper flakes, if desired.
- Place a lid on the pot, allow the broth to come to a simmer, then turn down to medium-low. Let the pot simmer for at least 30 minutes, or longer if desired. Taste the greens and adjust the salt, pepper, or sugar if needed (if your broth is low-sodium, you may want to add salt at this time). Serve the greens with a slotted spoon to leave the excess broth behind.

### *Nutrition Info*

Calories: 60.73kcal, Carbohydrates: 8.6g, Protein: 2.38g, Fat: 2.73g, Sodium: 311.73mg, Fiber: 2.22g

# 27 VEGETABLE ENCHILADA CASSEROLE

Prep Time: 15 mins
Cook Time: 55 mins
Total Time: 1 hr 10 mins
Servings: 6

### *Ingredients*

- 12 small corn tortillas
- 1.5 cups shredded "taco blend" cheese
- 1 zucchini (about 3/4 lb.)
- 1 15oz. can black beans, drained
- 1 cup frozen corn kernels
- 1 4oz. can diced green chiles
- 1/2 bunch (3-4 each) green onions
- 1/4 bunch fresh cilantro (optional)
- 1/4 tsp salt

Enchilada Sauce

- 2 Tbsp cooking oil
- 2 Tbsp chili powder
- 2 Tbsp all-purpose flour
- 2 cups water
- 3 oz. tomato paste
- 1/2 tsp ground cumin
- 1/2 tsp garlic powder
- 1/4 tsp cayenne pepper

- 3/4 tsp salt

**Instructions**

- Cut the zucchini into small cubes. Rinse and drain the black beans. Slice the green onions (both green and white portions). Pull the cilantro leaves from the stems and give them a rough chop. Combine the zucchini, black beans, frozen corn kernels, green onions, cilantro, and diced green chiles in a bowl. Add 1/4 tsp salt and stir until evenly combined.
- To make the enchilada sauce, combine the oil, chili powder, and flour in a small sauce pot. Whisk them together over medium heat and allow it to begin to bubble. Let the mixture bubble while whisking for about one minute. Add the water, tomato paste, cumin, garlic, cayenne, and salt. Whisk until smooth. Heat the sauce until thick and bubbly (about 3-5 minutes).
- Preheat the oven to 350 degrees. Prepare a 9x9 casserole dish by coating lightly with non-stick spray. Spread a 1/2 cup of the sauce in the bottom of the dish. Arrange 1/3 of the tortillas over the sauce, followed by 1/3 of the vegetable mixture. Drizzle 1/2 cup of the sauce over the vegetables, then top with 1/2 cup cheese. Repeat these layers two more times, or until the vegetable mix, sauce, and cheese are gone.

- Bake the casserole for 40-45 minutes, or until the edges are bubbly and the cheese just begins to brown on top. Slice into six portions and top with extra green onions and cilantro, if desired.

**Nutrition Info**

Calories: 375.3kcal, Carbohydrates: 50.3g, Protein: 16.68g, Fat: 14.22g, Sodium: 978.73mg, Fiber: 13.5g

## 28 TRIPLE BERRY OATMEAL MUFFINS

Prep Time: 15 mins
Cook Time: 20 mins
Total Time: 35 mins
Servings: 8 large muffins

### *Ingredients*

MUFFINS

- 1 cup all-purpose flour
- 1/4 cup whole wheat flour
- 1 cup rolled oats
- 1/4 cup brown sugar
- 1/4 cup white sugar
- 1/2 tsp salt
- 1 Tbsp baking powder
- 1/4 tsp cinnamon
- 1 cup milk
- 1/4 cup cooking oil
- 2 large eggs
- 1 cup frozen berries

OAT CRUMBLE TOPPING

- 1/2 cup rolled oats
- 2 Tbsp butter, cold
- 2 Tbsp brown sugar

- 1/4 tsp cinnamon

## Instructions

- Prepare the oat crumble topping first, so it's ready to go on the muffins as soon as they're mixed. In a small bowl, combine the oats, butter, brown sugar, and cinnamon. Use your hands to massage the oats, brown sugar, and cinnamon, into the butter until it's evenly combined and clumpy. Refrigerate the mixture until you're ready to top the muffins.
- Preheat the oven to 500ºF. In a large bowl, combine the all-purpose and whole wheat flours, oats, brown sugar, white sugar, salt, baking powder, and cinnamon. Stir well.
- In a separate bowl, whisk together the milk, eggs, and oil.
- Pour the whisked wet ingredients into the bowl with the dry ingredients. Stir just until they are combined, it doesn't need to be perfectly mixed. There may still be clumps and a few dry spots, but it's important to avoid over mixing.
- Add the frozen berries to the mixture and gently fold in. Again, avoid over mixing because the berry juice will turn the muffins blueish grey.
- Line eight muffin tin cups with paper liners, then fill each one to the top with the muffin batter (use more cups if needed, just make sure to fill

to the top). Sprinkle the prepared oat crumble topping onto each muffin.
- Transfer the muffin tin to the oven and immediately turn the heat down to 400ºF. Bake for 22-25 minutes, or until the muffins have risen into peaks, have cracked slightly, and are deep golden brown on top. Remove the muffins from the oven and the muffin tin (use a knife to loosen any parts that have spilled out over top) and allow them to cool.

### *Nutrition Info*

Calories: 320.54kcal, Carbohydrates: 45.18g, Protein: 7.06g, Fat: 13.69g, Sodium: 359.94mg, Fiber: 3.08g

# 29 CABBAGE AND CRANBERRY SALAD

Prep Time: 10 mins
Total Time: 10 mins
Servings: 4

## Ingredients

- 1/2 head purple cabbage
- 1/3 cup dried cranberries
- 1/4 cup sunflower seeds
- 2 oz. feta, crumbled
- 1/4 cup champagne vinaigrette

## Instructions

- Thinly slice or shred the cabbage.
- Combine the cabbage, cranberries, sunflower seeds, feta, and dressing in a large bowl. Stir until everything is well coated in dressing. Eat immediately or refrigerate until ready to eat.

## Nutrition Info

Calories: 205.73kcal, Carbohydrates: 23.4g, Protein: 6.13g, Fat: 11.23g, Sodium: 304.55mg, Fiber: 5.7g

## 30 CREAMY PESTO MAC AND CHEESE WITH SPINACH

Prep Time: 15 mins
Cook Time: 15 mins
Total Time: 30 mins
Servings: 6 (1 cup each)

### Ingredients

- 2 cups uncooked macaroni
- 2 Tbsp butter
- 2 Tbsp flour
- 2 cups whole milk
- 1/2 cup grated Romano or Parmesan
- 1/4 cup basil pesto
- 1/2 tsp salt
- Freshly cracked pepper
- 1/2 lb. frozen spinach

### Instructions

- Thaw the spinach at room temperature or in the microwave. Squeeze out the excess water. Set the spinach aside. Bring a large pot of water to a boil, then add the macaroni noodles. Boil for 7-10 minutes, or until al dente. Drain the macaroni in a colander.

- While the pasta is boiling, prepare the sauce. Add the butter and flour to a small sauce pot. Heat and stir the butter and flour over medium heat until it forms a creamy paste and begins to bubble. Continue to stir and cook for about one minute more.
- Whisk the milk into the butter and flour, then allow it to come up to a simmer, while whisking. When it reaches a simmer, the sauce will thicken. Remove the sauce from the heat.
- Whisk the Romano (or Parmesan) and pesto into the sauce until smooth. This will further thicken the sauce. Season the sauce with salt and freshly cracked pepper. Make sure the sauce is well seasoned as the flavors will be less concentrated once the pasta and spinach are stirred in.
- Return the cooked and drained pasta to the large pot (heat turned off) and add the thawed spinach. Pour the sauce over top, then stir until everything is combined and coated in sauce. Serve immediately.

### *Nutrition Info*

Calories: 333.58kcal, Carbohydrates: 39.75g, Protein: 12.33g, Fat: 14.08g, Sodium: 665.92mg, Fiber: 2.75g

# 31 BANANA NUT BREAKFAST FARRO

Prep Time: 5 mins
Cook Time: 3 mins
Total Time: 8 mins
Servings: 8

## *Ingredients*

- 1/2 cup cooked farro
- 1/2 cup milk (dairy, soy, or almond)
- 1/4 tsp vanilla extract
- 1/2 tsp brown sugar, maple syrup, or honey
- 1 banana
- 2 Tbsp chopped walnuts

## *Instructions*

- Add the cooked farro and milk to a bowl. Microwave on high for one minute (watching to prevent overflow) then stir. Cook for 2 minutes more, in 30 second intervals, stirring in between. After 3 minutes total, the farro should have absorbed some of the milk, be softer in texture, and the milk slightly more starchy and thick.
- Stir in the vanilla extract and sweetener (brown sugar, maple syrup, or honey).

- Slice the banana and place it on top. Sprinkle the chopped walnuts over the bowl, and enjoy.

**Nutrition Info**

Calories: 391.3kcal, Carbohydrates: 59.4g, Protein: 9.8g, Fat: 13.9g, Sodium: 71.8mg, Fiber: 6.1g

## 32 FRESH APPLE PIE SCONES

Prep Time: 15 mins
Cook Time: 20 mins
Total Time: 35 mins
Servings: 8

### *Ingredients*

SCONES

- 1 large egg
- 1/4 cup unsweetened apple sauce
- 1 tsp lemon juice
- 1 Tbsp sugar
- 1 medium apple
- 2 cups all-purpose flour (plus a small amount for dusting)
- 1/2 tsp salt
- 2 tsp baking powder
- 1 tsp cinnamon
- 1/2 tsp ground ginger
- 5 Tbsp cold butter

CINNAMON GLAZE (optional)

- 1/2 cup powdered sugar
- 1/2 tsp cinnamon
- 2 tsp water

## Instructions

- Preheat the oven to 400ºF. Wash the apple, cut it into quarters, then cut off the core from each piece. Use a box grater or large holed cheese grater to shred the apple.
- In a medium bowl, whisk together the egg, apple sauce, lemon juice, sugar, and shredded apple.
- In a separate large bowl, stir together the flour, salt, baking powder, cinnamon, and ginger. Once combined, add the butter and work it into the flour until it resembles coarse, damp sand.
- Finally, pour the bowl containing the apple egg mixture into the large bowl with the flour and butter. Stir just until a dough forms and no more dry flour remains on the bottom of the bowl.
- Turn the dough out onto a lightly floured surface and shape into a 6-8 inch wide, 1.5 inch thick disc (sprinkle more flour on your hands and on the surface of the dough if needed. The dough may be slightly sticky). Cut the disc into eight wedges.
- Line a baking sheet with parchment paper and place the cut scones on top. Bake the scones for 18-20 minutes in the fully preheated oven, or until they are just slightly golden brown on top. Allow the scones to cool completely.

- To make the glaze, stir together the powdered sugar, cinnamon, and water until a thick paste forms. Once the scones are fully cooled, drizzle the glaze over top.

***Nutrition Info***

Calories: 239.08kcal, Carbohydrates: 37.73g, Protein: 4.19g, Fat: 8.16g, Sodium: 304.68mg, Fiber: 1.76g

## 33 EGGS FLORENTINE BREAKFAST PIZZA

Prep Time: 15 mins
Cook Time: 15 mins
Total Time: 30 mins
Servings: 3 (2 slices each)

### Ingredients

White Sauce

- 1 Tbsp butter
- 1 Tbsp all-purpose flour
- 1 cup whole milk
- 1/8 tsp garlic powder
- 1/4 tsp salt

Pizza

- 1 pizza dough
- 1/4 lb. frozen spinach, thawed
- 1 cup shredded mozzarella
- 4 large eggs
- Freshly cracked pepper
- 1/2 Tbsp cornmeal (for pizza pan--optional)

### Instructions

- Adjust your oven rack to the highest level. Begin to preheat the oven to 500ºF.
- To make the white sauce, combine the butter and flour in a small sauce pot. Heat the butter and flour over medium-low heat, while whisking, until it begins to simmer. Simmer and whisk the mixture for about one minute.
- Whisk the milk into the butter and flour mixture. Allow it to come up to a simmer again, whisking often. When it reaches a simmer, it will thicken. Turn off the heat and whisk in the garlic and salt. Set the sauce aside to cool (it will thicken further as it cools).
- Prepare a 12-inch pizza pan with non-stick spray and/or cornmeal. Stretch the pizza dough out to cover the surface of the pizza pan. Pour the white sauce over the surface and spread it out with the back of a spoon. Bake the crust with the sauce for 5 minutes.
- Squeeze any excess moisture out of the spinach, then sprinkle the spinach over the surface of the par-baked pizza crust and sauce, followed by half of the mozzarella. Crack the four eggs onto the pizza, equally spaced around the surface. Add a small amount of freshly cracked pepper, then top the remainder of the mozzarella.
- Bake the pizza for 10-12 minutes, or until the cheese and crust are golden brown and the eggs are mostly set. Allow the pizza to cool for five

minutes before slicing (the eggs will continue to firm up after it comes out of the oven).

**Nutrition Info**

Calories: 753.97kcal, Carbohydrates: 94.07g, Protein: 30.07g, Fat: 25.5g, Sodium: 1679mg, Fiber: 3.83g

## 34 OVEN ROASTED FROZEN BROCCOLI

Prep Time: 5 mins
Cook Time: 30 mins
Total Time: 35 mins
Servings: 2 to 3 servings

### *Ingredients*

- 1/2 lb. frozen broccoli florets
- 1 Tbsp olive oil
- 1/2 Tbsp Montreal steak seasoning

### *Instructions*

- Preheat the oven to 400ºF. Line a baking sheet with parchment paper. Spread the frozen florets out over the baking sheet (no need to thaw).
- Drizzle the olive oil over the florets, then sprinkle the Montreal steak seasoning over top. Toss the florets in the oil and seasoning until everything is evenly distributed (it's okay if a lot of it falls onto the baking sheet, it will be stirred and redistributed again later).
- Transfer the baking sheet to the oven and roast for 20 minutes. Take the baking sheet out and use a spatula to stir the broccoli and redistribute the oil and spices. Return the baking sheet to the oven and roast for another 10 minutes, or until

the broccoli develops the amount of brownness desired. Serve hot.

**Nutrition Info**

Calories: 89kcal, Carbohydrates: 5.45g, Protein: 3.2g, Fat: 7.1g, Sodium: 402.45mg, Fiber: 3.4g

# 35 EASY HOMEMADE CORNBREAD RECIPE

Prep Time: 10 mins
Cook Time: 20 mins
Total Time: 30 mins
Servings: 8

## *Ingredients*

- 1 cup yellow cornmeal
- 1 cup all-purpose flour
- 1/4 cup sugar
- 4 tsp baking powder
- 1/2 tsp salt
- 1 cup milk
- 1 large egg
- 1/4 cup cooking oil

## *Instructions*

- Preheat the oven to 425 degrees and coat the inside of a 9-inch pie plate, cast iron skillet, or 8x8 casserole dish with non-stick spray (or butter for more flavor).
- In a large bowl, stir together the cornmeal, flour, sugar, baking powder, and salt until evenly combined.
- In a separate bowl, whisk together the milk, egg, and oil.

- Pour the bowl of wet ingredients into the bowl of dry ingredients and stir just until everything is moist. Avoid over stirring. It's okay if there are a few lumps.
- Pour the batter into the prepared dish and bake for about 20 minutes, or until the top and edges are golden brown. Cut into 8 pieces and serve.

### Nutrition Info

Calories: 241.23kcal, Carbohydrates: 35.39g, Protein: 4.79g, Fat: 9.15g, Sodium: 352.61mg, Fiber: 1.19g

# 36 POOR MAN'S BURRITO BOWLS

Prep Time: 5 mins
Cook Time: 20 mins
Total Time: 25 mins
Servings: 4

## *Ingredients*

- 2 cups uncooked long grain white rice
- 1/2 tsp salt
- 2 15oz. cans black beans
- 1/2 tsp ground cumin
- 1/4 tsp garlic powder
- 1 16oz. jar salsa
- 6 oz. shredded cheese
- 1 bunch green onions
- 1 jalapeño (optional)

## *Instructions*

- Add the rice, salt, and 3 cups water to a medium sauce pot. Place a lid on top, turn the heat on to high, and allow the water to come up to a full boil. Once boiling, turn the heat down to low and let it continue to simmer for 15 minutes. After 15 minutes, turn the heat off and let it sit, with the lid in place, for an additional five minutes. Fluff just before serving.

- While the rice is cooking, make the beans. Add both cans of black beans (undrained) to a small sauce pot, along with the cumin, and garlic powder. Heat over medium, stirring often, until heated through.
- Slice the green onions and jalapeño (if using).
- Once the rice is cooked, build the bowls. Add one cup cooked rice, 1/2 cup warm black beans, 1/3 cup salsa, and 1 oz. shredded cheese (about 1/4 cup) to each bowl. Top with a few sliced green onions and jalapeños, then serve.

**Nutrition Info**

Calories: 521.75kcal, Carbohydrates: 85.28g, Protein: 20.32g, Fat: 10.32g, Sodium: 1078.75mg, Fiber: 15.22g

# 37 ROASTED RED PEPPER HUMMUS WRAPS

Prep Time: 20 mins
Total Time: 20 mins
Servings: 6

## Ingredients

HUMMUS

- 1 15oz. can chickpeas
- 1/4 cup lemon juice
- 1/4 cup tahini
- 2 Tbsp olive oil
- 1/4 tsp ground cumin
- 1/4 tsp garlic powder
- 1/2 tsp salt
- 1/4 cup water

WRAP

- 1/2 12oz. jar roasted red peppers
- 1 cucumber
- 3 oz. feta
- 6 pitas
- 6 cups baby spinach or baby greens

## Instructions

- To make the hummus, drain the chickpeas and add them to a food processor along with the lemon juice, tahini, olive oil, cumin, garlic powder, and salt. Pulse until the mixture is crumbly, then slowly add up to 1/4 cup water until the mixture is smooth and fluffy.
- Remove the red peppers from the jar and slice them thinly. Cut the feta into 1/2 oz. cubes. Thinly slice the cucumbers.
- Spread about 1/4 cup hummus inside or over the surface of a pita. Add a few roasted red pepper strips, one of the feta cubes (crumbled), some sliced cucumber, and a cup or so of baby spinach. Fold up the sides of the pita and eat!

**Nutrition Info**

Calories: 495.37kcal, Carbohydrates: 70.27g, Protein: 17.5g, Fat: 16.32g, Sodium: 1114.87mg, Fiber: 8.25g

# 38 MEDITERRANEAN FARRO SALAD WITH SPICED CHICKPEAS

Prep Time: 15 mins
Cook Time: 5 mins
Total Time: 20 mins
Servings: 4

## *Ingredients*

DRESSING

- 1/3 cup tahini
- 1/3 cup water
- 1/4 cup lemon juice
- 2 cloves garlic, minced
- 1/2 tsp ground cumin
- 1/4 tsp cayenne pepper
- 1/2 tsp salt

SPICED CHICKPEAS

- 1 15oz. can chickpeas
- 1 Tbsp olive oil
- 1/2 tsp smoked paprika
- 1/4 tsp garlic powder
- 1/8 tsp cayenne pepper (optional)
- Freshly cracked black pepper (10-15 cranks of a mill)

- Salt to taste

SALAD

- 3 cups cooked farro (or other grain)
- 2 Roma tomatoes
- 1 cucumber
- 1/4 bunch fresh parsley

***Instructions***

- To make the dressing, combine the tahini, water, lemon juice, minced garlic, cumin, cayenne, and salt in a blender. Blend until smooth. Set the dressing aside until ready to use (keep in the refrigerator for up to 5 days).
- Rinse and drain the chickpeas in a colander. Heat the olive oil in a non-stick skillet over medium heat. Once hot add the drained chick peas. Sprinkle the smoked paprika, garlic powder, cayenne pepper (if using), and some freshly cracked pepper over top. Stir the chickpeas to coat in the spices, then continue to sauté for about five minutes, or until the outside of the chickpeas are slightly browned and blistered. Season with salt to taste.
- Chop the tomatoes, cucumber, and parsley. Place about 3/4 cup cooked farro in each bowl, then top with chopped tomato, chopped

cucumber, spiced chickpeas, and a large pinch of chopped parsley. Drizzle the dressing over top and serve.

### Nutrition Info

Calories: 467.88kcal, Carbohydrates: 64.38g, Protein: 16.4g, Fat: 18.53g, Sodium: 889.9mg, Fiber: 13.3g

## 39 VEGETARIAN SHEPHERD'S PIE

Prep Time: 10 mins
Cook Time: 45 mins
Total Time: 55 mins
Servings: 6

### *Ingredients*

- 1 cup cooked lentils (optional)
- 2 cloves garlic
- 1 yellow onion
- 1 Tbsp olive oil
- 3 carrots
- 2 ribs celery
- 8 oz. button mushrooms
- 3/4 tsp salt
- 1 tsp dried thyme
- 1/2 tsp smoked paprika
- Freshly cracked pepper
- 1 Tbsp tomato paste
- 1 Tbsp flour
- 1 cup vegetable broth
- 1 cup frozen peas
- 4 cups mashed potatoes

### *Instructions*

- Mince the garlic and dice the onion. Sauté the onion and garlic with olive oil in a large skillet over medium heat until the onions are soft and transparent (3-5 minutes).
- While the onions and garlic are cooking, peel and dice the carrots, dice the celery, and slice the mushrooms. Once the onions are soft, add the carrots and celery to the skillet and continue to sauté until the celery begins to soften slightly (5 minutes).
- Finally, add the mushrooms, salt, thyme, smoked paprika, and freshly cracked pepper to the skillet. Continue to sauté until the mushrooms have fully softened (3-5 minutes). Add the tomato paste and flour to the skillet. Stir and cook the vegetables with the flour and tomato paste until the vegetables are coated and the pasty mixture begins to coat the bottom of the skillet (about 2 minutes).
- Add the vegetable broth to the skillet, stirring to dissolve the flour and tomato paste from the bottom of the skillet. Allow the broth to come up to a simmer, at which point it will become slightly thicker. Stir in the cooked lentils and frozen peas, and allow to mixture to heat through.
- Preheat the oven to 400ºF. Pour the vegetable mixture into a casserole dish, or use your skillet if it is oven safe. Spread the mashed potatoes out

over the surface of the vegetables and gravy. Use your spoon to make a decorative pattern in the mashed potatoes, if desired.
- Bake the shepherd's pie in the fully preheated oven for 15 minutes, or until everything is heated through. To achieve a browned surface on the mashed potatoes (optional), turn on the oven's broiler (and place the pie under it, if not already), and watch closely until the top has browned to your liking.

**Nutrition Info**

Calories: 103.13kcal, Carbohydrates: 16.3g, Protein: 5.13g, Fat: 2.78g, Sodium: 507.77mg, Fiber: 4.82g

## 40 5 MINUTE NACHO CHEESE SAUCE

Cook Time: 5 mins
Total Time: 5 mins
Servings: 6 (1/4 cup each)

### *Ingredients*

- 2 Tbsp butter
- 2 Tbsp flour
- 1 cup whole milk
- 6 oz. medium cheddar, shredded (about 1.5 cups)
- 1/4 tsp salt
- 1/4 tsp chili powder

### *Instructions*

- Add the butter and flour to a small sauce pot. Heat and whisk the butter and flour together until they become bubbly and foamy. Continue to cook and whisk the bubbly mixture for about 60 seconds.
- Whisk the milk into the flour and butter mixture. Turn the heat up slightly and allow the milk to come to a simmer while whisking. When it reaches a simmer, the mixture will thicken. Once it's thick enough to coat a spoon, turn off the heat.

- Stir in the shredded cheddar, one handful at a time, until melted into the sauce. If needed, place the pot over a low flame to help the cheese melt. Do not over heat the cheese sauce.
- Once all the cheese is melted into the sauce, stir in the salt and chili powder. Taste and adjust the seasoning as needed. If the sauce becomes too thick, simply whisk in an additional splash of milk.

## Nutrition Info

Calories: 183.1kcal, Carbohydrates: 4.92g, Protein: 8.13g, Fat: 14.65g, Sodium: 337.23mg, Fiber: 0.32g

## 41 CARAMELIZED BANANA AND PEANUT BUTTER QUESADILLA

Prep Time: 5 mins
Cook Time: 10 mins
Total Time: 15 mins
Servings: 1

### Ingredients

- 1 ripe banana
- 1 small flour tortilla
- 1 Tbsp peanut butter
- 1/2 Tbsp butter
- 1/2 Tbsp brown sugar
- 1 dash cinnamon

### Instructions

- Slice the banana. Melt the butter in a small skillet over medium heat. Once melted, add the sliced banana and brown sugar. Cook the banana in the butter and brown sugar until the slices turn golden brown and slightly sticky. Remove the skillet from the heat.
- Spread the peanut butter over half of the quesadilla. Scoop the caramelized banana slices onto the peanut butter. Sprinkle a dash of

cinnamon on top. Fold the empty half of the tortilla over the filled side.
- Place the quesadilla in a clean dry skillet and cook over medium heat until golden brown and crispy on both sides. Slice the quesadilla into triangles using a large knife or pizza cutter, then serve.

**Nutrition Info**

Calories: 397.5kcal, Carbohydrates: 58.6g, Protein: 7.9g, Fat: 17.1g, Sodium: 360.3mg, Fiber: 6g

# 42 EASY SPINACH RICOTTA PASTA

Prep Time: 10 mins
Cook Time: 20 mins
Total Time: 30 mins
Servings: 4

## *Ingredients*

- 1/2 lb. uncooked fettuccine
- 2 Tbsp olive oil
- 2 cloves garlic
- 1/2 cup milk
- 1 cup whole milk ricotta
- 1/4 tsp salt
- Freshly cracked pepper
- 1/4 lb. frozen chopped spinach

## *Instructions*

- Place the frozen spinach in a colander to thaw while you work on the pasta and sauce.
- Bring a large pot of water to a boil and then add the pasta. Let the pasta boil until al dente, then drain in a colander. Reserve about 1/2 cup of the pasta cooking water to help loosen the sauce later if needed.
- While the pasta is boiling, prepare the ricotta sauce. Mince the garlic and add it to a large

skillet with the olive oil. Cook over medium-low heat for 1-2 minutes, or just until soft and fragrant (but not browned). Add the milk and ricotta, then stir until relatively smooth (the ricotta may be slightly grainy). Allow the sauce to heat through and come to a low simmer. The sauce will thicken slightly as it simmers. Once it's thick enough to coat the spoon (3-5 minutes), season with salt and pepper.

- Squeeze the thawed spinach to remove as much excess water as possible (squeeze it in your fist), then add it to the ricotta sauce. Stir until the spinach is distributed throughout the sauce. Taste and adjust salt or pepper if needed. Turn the heat off.
- Add the cooked and drained pasta to the sauce and toss to coat. If the sauce becomes to thick or dry, add a small amount of the reserved pasta cooking water. Serve warm.

### *Nutrition Info*

Calories: 403.7kcal, Carbohydrates: 49.95g, Protein: 14.45g, Fat: 16.3g, Sodium: 362.4mg, Fiber: 2.68g

## 43 EASY HOT AND SOUR SOUP WITH VEGETABLES AND TOFU

Prep Time: 20 mins
Cook Time: 15 mins
Total Time: 35 mins
Servings: 4

### *Ingredients*

- 1 Tbsp canola oil
- 1 Tbsp grated fresh ginger
- 4 green onions
- 1/4 red cabbage
- 3 carrots
- 8 oz. button mushrooms
- 6 cups vegetable broth
- 1/2 Tbsp soy sauce (or more to taste)
- 1.5-2 Tbsp rice vinegar
- 1 Tbsp chili garlic sauce or sambal olek
- 14 oz. block extra firm tofu

### Instructions

- Thinly slice the cabbage, mushrooms, and the green onions (both the green and white ends of the onions). Peel the carrots, then either slice them thinly, use a vegetable peeler to slice them

into ribbons, or cut them into thin sticks (julienne).
- Add the canola oil, grated ginger, and the sliced white ends of the green onion to a large pot. Sauté the ginger and onion over medium heat until soft (1-2 minutes). Add the vegetable broth to the pot, along with the soy sauce, vinegar, and chili garlic sauce. The amount of soy sauce, vinegar, and chili garlic sauce needed may be subjective and will depend on how much salt your vegetable broth contains. Start with a smaller amount of each, then add more to your taste. The final broth should be tangy and spicy. Heat the broth until piping hot.
- Drain the tofu, then cut it into small cubes (small enough to fit on a spoon). Add the tofu to the hot broth, and allow it to heat through ( a few minutes).
- Either add the sliced vegetables to the soup pot and cook until softened, or divide the vegetables into individual bowls for serving, then spoon the hot broth over top. Sprinkle the sliced green portion of the green onions over each bow. More chili garlic sauce can also be added to each bowl if desired.

### *Nutrition Info*

Calories: 131.5kcal, Carbohydrates: 13.05g, Protein: 9.12g, Fat: 5.72g, Sodium: 1068mg, Fiber: 3.28g

# 44 SPINACH AND CHICKPEA RICE PILAF

Prep Time: 10 mins
Cook Time: 30 mins
Total Time: 40 mins
Servings: 4 1.25 cups each

## *Ingredients*

- 1 fresh lemon
- 1/2 lb. frozen chopped spinach
- 2 cloves garlic
- 1 yellow onion
- 2 Tbsp olive oil
- 1 cup long grain white rice (uncooked)
- 1 tsp smoked paprika
- 1/2 tsp dried oregano
- 1/4 tsp ground cumin
- 1 15oz. can chickpeas
- 1 3/4 cup vegetable broth
- 1 oz. feta, crumbled
- 1 pinch crushed red pepper (optional)

## *Instructions*

- Zest the lemon, set the zest aside, then squeeze the juice into a small bowl. Thaw the spinach in the microwave and then squeeze out the excess liquid.

- Mince the garlic and dice the onion. Sauté the onion and garlic in olive oil over medium heat in a deep skillet until the onion is soft and translucent (about 3-5 minutes).
- Add the smoked paprika, oregano, cumin, and dry rice to the skillet. Stir and cook over medium heat for about 2 minutes to toast the rice and spices. You should hear the rice popping and it should begin to look slightly translucent.
- Drain the chickpeas and add them to the skillet along with the spinach. Add about 2 Tbsp of the lemon juice and the vegetable broth to the skillet, then stir the ingredients to combine.
- Place a lid on the skillet and turn the heat up to medium-high. Allow it to come to a boil, then immediately turn it down to low or just above low. Let the skillet continue to simmer for 15 minutes, with the lid in place. After 15 minutes, turn the heat off and let it sit undisturbed for an additional 5 minutes.
- Remove the lid and fluff the skillet with a fork to redistribute the chickpeas and spinach. Sprinkle the lemon zest and crumbled feta over the skillet just before serving.

### *Nutrition Info*

Calories: 268.6kcal, Carbohydrates: 41.4g, Protein: 8.5g, Fat: 8.2g, Sodium: 554.5mg, Fiber: 5.3g

## 45 HOMEMADE NAAN BREAD RECIPE

Prep Time: 1 hr 30 mins
Cook Time: 25 mins
Total Time: 1 hr 55 mins
Servings: 8

### *Ingredients*

- 2 tsp dry active yeast
- 1 tsp sugar
- 1/2 cup water
- 2 1/2-3 cups flour, divided
- 1/2 tsp salt
- 1/4 cup olive oil
- 1/3 cup plain yogurt
- 1 large egg

### *Instructions*

- In a small bowl, combine the yeast, sugar and water. Stir to dissolve then let sit for a few minutes or until it is frothy on top. Once frothy, whisk in the oil, yogurt, and egg until evenly combined.
- In a separate medium bowl, combine 1 cup of the flour with the salt. Next, pour the bowl of wet ingredients to the flour/salt mixture and stir until well combined. Continue adding flour, a

half cup at a time, until you can no longer stir it with a spoon (about 1 to 1.5 cups later).
- At that point, turn the ball of dough out onto a lightly floured surface and knead the ball of dough for about 3 minutes, adding small amounts of flour as necessary to keep the dough from sticking. You'll end up using between 2.5 to 3 cups flour total. The dough should be smooth and very soft but not sticky. Avoid adding excessive amounts of flour as you knead, as this can make the dough too dry and stiff.
- Loosely cover the dough and let it rise until double in size (about 1 hour). After it rises, gently flatten the dough into a disc and cut it into 8 equal pieces. Shape each piece into a small ball.
- Heat a large, heavy bottomed skillet over medium heat. Working with one ball at a time, roll it out until it is about 1/4 inch thick or approximately 6 inches in diameter. Place the rolled out dough onto the hot skillet and cook until the bottom is golden brown and large bubbles have formed on the surface (see photos below). Flip the dough and cook the other side until golden brown as well. Stack the cooked flat bread on a plate and cover with a towel to keep warm as you cook the remaining pieces. Serve plain or brushed with melted butter and sprinkled with herbs!

**Nutrition Info**

Calories: 250.81kcal, Carbohydrates: 37.23g, Protein: 6.36g, Fat: 8.18g, Sodium: 161.29mg, Fiber: 1.54g

## 46 PINEAPPLE SRIRACHA BREAKFAST BOWLS

Prep Time: 5 mins
Cook Time: 5 mins
Total Time: 10 mins

### Ingredients

- 1 cup cooked rice (preferably jasmine rice)
- 1 tsp soy sauce
- 1 tsp sriracha
- Splash of sesame oil
- 1/3 cup chopped pineapple
- 1 green onion, sliced
- 1 large egg
- Salt and pepper to taste

### Instructions

- Reheat the cooked rice in the microwave, then season with soy sauce, sriracha, and a splash of sesame oil.
- Roughly chop the pineapple pieces and thinly slice the green onion. Stir them into the seasoned rice.
- Fry the egg, seasoning it with salt and pepper, and leaving the yolk slightly runny. Top the seasoned rice bowl with the egg and enjoy.

*Nutrition Info*

Calories: 359.5kcal, Carbohydrates: 54.5g, Protein: 11.5g, Fat: 9.5g, Sodium: 1479.2mg, Fiber: 1.9g

## 47 CHILI ROASTED SWEET POTATOES

Prep Time: 10 mins
Cook Time: 45 mins
Total Time: 55 mins
Servings: 4

### Ingredients

- 2 lbs. sweet potatoes
- 1 Tbsp chili powder
- 2 Tbsp olive oil
- 1/4 tsp salt (or to taste)

### Instructions

- Preheat the oven to 400ºF. Line a baking sheet with aluminum foil.
- Wash and peel the sweet potatoes, then cut them into 1/2 inch cubes. Place the cubed sweet potatoes into a large bowl and drizzle with the olive oil, chili powder, and salt. Toss the potatoes until evenly coated in oil and spices.
- Spread the seasoned sweet potatoes out over the prepared baking sheet so they are in a single layer. Roast the potatoes in the preheated oven for 45 minutes, stirring once half way through. After 45 minutes, the sweet potatoes should be soft and slightly browned on the edges. Total

cooking time will ultimately depend on the size of your cubes.

**Nutrition Info**

Calories: 260.8kcal, Carbohydrates: 46.78g, Protein: 3.85g, Fat: 7.15g, Sodium: 330mg, Fiber: 7.53g

## 48 CREAMY SPINACH ARTICHOKE PIZZA

Prep Time: 12 hrs
Cook Time: 25 mins
Total Time: 12 hrs 25 mins
Servings: 3 (2 slices each)

### *Ingredients*

DOUGH

- 2 cups all-purpose flour
- 1 tsp salt
- 1/8 tsp instant yeast
- 1 Tbsp olive oil
- 3/4-1 cup water

CREAMY SPINACH SAUCE

- 1/2 lb. frozen chopped spinach
- 1 Tbsp butter
- 1 clove garlic
- 4 oz. cream cheese
- 1/2 cup milk
- 1/4 tsp salt

PIZZA

- 1 Tbsp cooking oil

- 1/2 15oz. can artichoke hearts
- 1 pinch crushed red pepper (optional)
- 1 cup shredded mozzarella

**Instructions**

- Begin the dough the night before. In a large bowl stir together the flour, salt, and yeast. Combine the olive oil and 3/4 cup water, then pour it into the bowl with the flour. Stir until a single (slightly wet and sticky) ball of dough forms with no dry flour left on the bottom of the bowl. Add one to two tablespoons more of water, if needed, to form a ball of dough. Loosely cover the dough and let it sit at room temperature for 12-18 hours.
- The next day let the spinach thaw and then squeeze out as much moisture as possible. Preheat the oven to 450ºF and pour 1 Tbsp of cooking oil into a 10 or 12-inch cast iron skillet. Spread the oil around the skillet, including up the side walls.
- To make the sauce, mince the garlic and add it to a small pot along with the butter. Sauté the butter and garlic for 1-2 minutes over medium-low heat, or until the garlic is soft and fragrant. Add the cream cheese, milk, and salt to the butter and garlic. Whisk and cook over medium-low heat until the cream cheese has melted into

the milk and a thick sauce forms (3-5 minutes). Finally, stir the squeeze-dried spinach into the sauce, breaking up any clumps as you stir. Remove the sauce from the heat and set aside.

- Use the excess oil from the skillet to coat your hands, then scrape the fermented dough out of the bowl. Gently press and stretch the loose dough into the skillet until it evenly covers the bottom.
- Spread the creamy spinach sauce over the dough, covering from edge to edge. Drain the artichoke hearts, give them a rough chop, then sprinkle over the creamy spinach sauce. Add a pinch of red pepper flakes, if desired. Finally, top the pizza with the shredded mozzarella.
- Bake the pizza in the fully preheated oven for 20-25 minutes, or until the edges are sizzling and the top is golden brown. Remove the pizza from the oven and slide a butter knife around the edges to loosen any melted cheese. Either slide the whole pizza onto a cutting board or carefully slice the pizza in the pan. Cut into six slices and serve.

### *Nutrition Info*

Calories: 794.33kcal, Carbohydrates: 88.07g, Protein: 27.7g, Fat: 37.67g, Sodium: 1864.57mg, Fiber: 12.87g

## 49 SMOKY TOMATO SOUP

Prep Time: 10 mins
Cook Time: 20 mins
Total Time: 30 mins
Servings: 4 (1.25 cups each)

### *Ingredients*

- 2 Tbsp olive oil
- 1 small yellow onion
- 2 cloves garlic
- 2 Tbsp tomato paste
- 1/2 Tbsp smoked paprika
- 1/2 tsp cumin
- 2 15oz. cans fire roasted diced tomatoes
- 1 cup vegetable broth
- 1/2 tsp brown sugar
- Freshly cracked pepper to taste

### *Instructions*

- Finely dice the onion and mince the garlic. Add them to a soup pot with the olive oil and cook over medium heat until the onions are soft and translucent.
- Add the tomato paste, smoked paprika, and cumin to the pot. Continue to stir and cook for

about two minutes to slightly caramelize the tomato paste and toast the spices.
- Add the cans of fire roasted tomatoes, vegetable broth, brown sugar, and some freshly cracked pepper. Stir to combine and heat through (about 10 minutes). Taste and adjust the seasoning if needed (salt may be needed depending on the brand of broth used).

**Nutrition Info**

Calories: 136.7kcal, Carbohydrates: 16.1g, Protein: 2.55g, Fat: 6.93g, Sodium: 617.43mg, Fiber: 4.58g

## 50 CHEDDAR GRITS BREAKFAST BOWLS

Prep Time: 10 mins
Cook Time: 20 mins
Total Time: 30 mins
Servings: 4

### *Ingredients*

- 4 cups water
- 1 tsp salt
- 1 cup quick cooking yellow grits
- 2 Tbsp butter
- 1/2 cup whole milk
- 4 oz medium cheddar, grated
- 4 large eggs
- 1 cup salsa
- 4 green onions, sliced
- Freshly cracked pepper

### *Instructions*

- Add the water and salt to a medium sauce pot. Place a lid on top, turn the heat on to high, and bring the water up to a rolling boil. Once boiling, stir in the grits. Turn the heat down to low, replace the lid, and let simmer for 5-7 minutes, or until thickened.*

- Add the butter and milk to the grits and stir until the butter has melted and the grits are smooth. Stir in the grated cheddar, one handful at a time, until fully melted in and smooth. Leave the lid on the pot with the burner turned off to keep the grits warm.
- Cook four eggs using your favorite method (fried, scrambled, soft boiled, etc.). Slice the green onions.
- To build the bowls, place one cup of the cheddar grits in a bowl, top with one egg, 1/4 cup salsa, some freshly cracked pepper, and a sprinkle of sliced green onions.

### *Nutrition Info*

Calories: 427.23kcal, Carbohydrates: 38.83g, Protein: 17.4g, Fat: 21.4g, Sodium: 1420.95mg, Fiber: 3.08g

# 51 GARDEN VEGETABLE QUINOA SOUP

Prep Time: 10 mins
Cook Time: 40 mins
Total Time: 50 mins
Servings: 8 (1.25 cup each)

## *Ingredients*

- 1 Tbsp olive oil
- 1 yellow onion
- 4 cloves garlic
- 3 carrots
- 3 ribs celery
- 1 15oz. can kidney beans
- 1 15oz. can fire roasted diced tomatoes
- 1/2 tsp dried basil
- 1 tsp dried oregano
- 1/2 tsp smoked paprika
- Freshly cracked black pepper
- 1 cup quinoa, uncooked
- 4 cups vegetable broth
- 2 cups water
- 1/4 lb. frozen spinach

## *Instructions*

- Mince the garlic and dice the onion. Add the olive oil, garlic, and onion to a large pot and

sauté over medium-low heat until the onions are soft and transparent.
- While the garlic and onion are cooking, wash and peel the carrots, then slice into 1/4-inch thick rounds. Wash the celery and slice into 1/4-inch pieces. Add the carrots and celery to the pot and continue to sauté until they just begin to soften (about 5 minutes).
- While the carrots and celery are cooking, rinse the quinoa well with cool running water in a wire mesh sieve. Drain and rinse the kidney beans. Add the quinoa, kidney beans, diced tomatoes (with juices), basil, oregano, smoked paprika, and some freshly cracked pepper (about 20 cranks of a pepper mill) to the pot.
- Add the vegetable broth and water to the pot, place a lid on top, and turn the heat up to medium-high. Allow the pot to come to a boil, then turn the heat down to low and let simmer for 25 minutes (make sure it's simmering the entire time, turning the heat up just slightly if it stops).
- After simmering for 25 minutes the quinoa should be slightly translucent and tender. If not, let simmer a few minutes longer. Stir in 1/4 lb. of frozen spinach until heated through. Taste the soup and add salt or adjust the seasonings if necessary. Serve hot.

**Nutrition Info**

Calories: 204.2kcal, Carbohydrates: 35.04g, Protein: 8.9g, Fat: 3.75g, Sodium: 716.56mg, Fiber: 6.68g

# 52 SAVORY VEGETARIAN STUFFING RECIPE

Prep Time: 20 mins
Cook Time: 1 hr 5 mins
Total Time: 1 hr 25 mins
Servings: 8 1 cup each

## Ingredients

- 8 oz mushrooms
- 4 stalks celery
- 3 carrots
- 1 yellow onion
- 4 cloves garlic
- 1/4 bunch parsley
- 6 Tbsp salted butter, divided
- 1 tsp dried sage
- 1 tsp dried thyme
- Freshly cracked pepper
- 1/4 tsp salt (or to taste)
- 1/2 cup chopped walnuts
- 1 large loaf French bread (stale*)
- 1.5 cups vegetable broth

## Instructions

- Begin by preparing the vegetables. Wash and slice the mushrooms, wash and dice the celery, peel and shred the carrots (use a large-holed

cheese grater), dice the onion, mince the garlic, and chop the parsley.
- Add 3 Tbsp of the butter to a large pot along with the sliced mushrooms. Sauté the mushrooms over medium heat until they have released all of their moisture and have begun to caramelize and brown on the edges (about 5-7 minutes).
- Add the garlic, onion, sage, thyme, some freshly cracked pepper, and 1/4 tsp salt to the pot. Continue to sauté the onions are soft and transparent (about 3-5 minutes), add the celery and continue to sauté for a few minutes more. Finally, add the shredded carrots and continue to sauté for a couple more minutes, or just until the carrots begin to soften.
- While sautéing the vegetables, add the chopped walnuts to a dry skillet. Cook and stir the walnut pieces over medium heat for 2-3 minutes, or just until they begin to give off a nutty aroma. Remove them from the heat immediately.
- Finally, add the toasted walnuts, the remaining 3 Tbsp butter, and a handful of fresh parsley to the pot. Stir until the butter has fully melted. Taste the vegetable mixture and add a touch more salt if needed. It should be well seasoned.
- Preheat the oven to 350ºF. Cut the stale bread into 1/2-inch cubes. Add the cubes to the pot with the sautéed vegetables and herbs. Stir well to coat the bread in the butter. Finally, pour in

the vegetable broth, 1/2 cup at a time, stirring well each time before adding more. The bread will not be completely saturated, but will absorb more moisture as the stuffing bakes.
- Coat the inside of a 3-quart casserole dish with non-stick spray. Add the stuffing mixture to the casserole dish, spread it out evenly, and compress it down slightly. Cover the dish with foil. Bake the stuffing in the preheated oven for 30 minutes, then remove the foil and bake for an additional 15 minutes, or until the top is golden brown and crispy. Garnish with any remaining chopped parsley just before serving.

### *Nutrition Info*

Calories: 316.41kcal, Carbohydrates: 38.33g, Protein: 8.89g, Fat: 14.41g, Sodium: 710.19mg, Fiber: 3.55g

# 53 CHILI GARLIC TOFU BOWLS

Prep Time: 30 mins
Cook Time: 30 mins
Total Time: 1 hr
Servings: 4

## Ingredients

SESAME KALE

- 1 bunch kale
- 1 Tbsp cooking oil
- 2 cloves garlic
- 1 Tbsp soy sauce
- 1 tsp toasted sesame oil
- 1 Tbsp sesame seeds

CHILI GARLIC TOFU

- 14 oz block firm tofu
- 2 Tbsp chili garlic sauce
- 1 Tbsp soy sauce
- 1 Tbsp brown sugar

BOWLS

- 4 cups cooked brown rice
- 1 lime

- 1/4 bunch cilantro (optional)

## *Instructions*

- Remove the tofu from its package and wrap it in a clean, lint-free kitchen towel or a few layers of paper towel. Place the wrapped tofu between two plates and place something heavy on top (like a pot full of water). Let the tofu press for at least 30 minutes.
- While the tofu is pressing, prepare the kale. Remove the stems from the kale, then cut the leaves into one-inch wide strips. Rinse the leaves well in a colander with cool water. Let drain.
- Mince the garlic and add it to large pot with one tablespoon cooking oil. Sauté over medium heat for about one minute. Add the washed kale and continue to stir and cook until the kale is wilted (about five minutes). Stir in the soy sauce, sesame oil, and sesame seeds. Set the kale aside.
- Prepare the sauce for the tofu. In a small bowl, stir together the chili garlic sauce, soy sauce, and brown sugar. Once the tofu is finished pressing, cut it into small cubes or rectangles.
- Heat a large skillet over medium-high heat. Once hot, add one tablespoon of cooking oil. Tilt the skillet to make sure the surface is completely covered. Add the tofu pieces. Let them fry until

golden brown on bottom, then flip and fry until golden brown on the other side. Continue until the pieces are golden brown on most sides. (The tofu will stick until it is browned, at which point it will loosen from the skillet, so don't try to move or flip the tofu pieces too early.)
- Once the tofu is browned on most sides, turn off the heat, pour the prepared chili garlic sauce into the skillet, and stir to coat. The sauce will thicken slightly and absorb into the tofu.
- To build the bowls, add one cup of cooked rice to each bowl along with 1/4 of the sesame kale and 1/4 of the chili garlic tofu pieces. Slice a lime into wedges and serve each bowl with one or two wedges and a few sprigs of fresh cilantro. Squeeze fresh lime juice over the bowl just before eating.

### *Nutrition Info*

Calories: 421.43kcal, Carbohydrates: 61.45g, Protein: 17.73g, Fat: 12.4g, Sodium: 1261.83mg, Fiber: 6.35g

# 54 ROASTED APPLE CRANBERRY RELISH

Prep Time: 10 mins
Cook Time: 55 mins
Total Time: 1 hr 5 mins
Servings: 4-6 cups

## *Ingredients*

- 12 oz bag fresh cranberries
- 3 medium apples* (about 1.5 lbs.)
- 1/2 cup brown sugar
- 1/2 tsp cinnamon
- 1/4 tsp ground cloves
- 1 tsp lemon juice

## *Instructions*

- Preheat the oven to 350ºF. Wash the cranberries and place them in a large 8x13-inch casserole dish (2-3 quart dish). Peel, core, and cut the apples into cubes roughly the same size as the cranberries. Place the cubed apples in the dish with the cranberries.
- To the apples and cranberries add the brown sugar, cinnamon, cloves, and lemon juice. Toss the ingredients together until well combined.
- Roast the fruit in the preheated oven for 45-55 minutes, or until it is a thick, jam-like

consistency. Stir the mixture once at 30 minutes, and again at 45 minutes to check doneness. Taste the relish and adjust the sugar or lemon juice if needed. Serve warm or refrigerate for later.

### *Nutrition Info*

Calories: 432.05kcal, Carbohydrates: 112.95g, Protein: 1.55g, Fat: 0.65g, Sodium: 22.4mg, Fiber: 13.15g

# 55 CREAMY MUSHROOM HERB PASTA

Prep Time: 5 mins
Cook Time: 25 mins
Total Time: 30 mins
Servings: 4

## Ingredients

- 8 oz mushrooms
- 12 oz fettuccine
- 2 cloves garlic, minced
- 3 Tbsp butter
- 3 Tbsp all-purpose flour
- 1.5 cups vegetable broth
- 3 sprigs fresh thyme (or 1/4 tsp dried)
- 1 tsp rubbed sage
- 1/2 cup half and half
- Salt and pepper to taste

## Instructions

- Wash the mushrooms to remove any dirt or debris, then thinly slice them.
- Begin cooking the fettuccine according to the package directions. Cook the pasta just until al dente, then drain in a colander. The pasta will continue to soften slightly once it's in the

creamy mushroom herb sauce, so do not overcook it.
- While the pasta is cooking, add the butter and minced garlic to a large skillet. Sauté the garlic over medium heat for 1-2 minutes, or just until fragrant and tender. Do not let the butter or garlic turn brown.
- Add the sliced mushrooms and continue to cook until the mushrooms have turned dark brown and all of the moisture they release has evaporated (5-7 minutes). Turn the heat down slightly to medium-low, add the flour, and continue to sauté until the flour begins to coat the bottom of the skillet and turns golden brown (about 2-3 minutes).
- Whisk the vegetable broth into the skillet with the flour and mushrooms. Whisk until all the flour has dissolved off the bottom of the skillet. Add the thyme, sage, and some freshly cracked pepper. Turn the heat up to medium and allow the sauce to come to a simmer, at which point it will thicken.
- Stir the half and half into the sauce and allow it to return to a gentle simmer. Taste the sauce and adjust the salt or pepper as needed (the amount of salt needed will depend on the type of broth used. I added approximately 1/4 tsp).
- Add the drained pasta to the sauce in the skillet. Toss to coat and allow the pasta to heat through

over medium-low heat. The pasta will absorb some of the liquid and flavors, and further thicken the sauce. Serve hot.

**Nutrition Info**

Calories: 472.45kcal, Carbohydrates: 73.5g, Protein: 14.55g, Fat: 13.28g, Sodium: 602.15mg, Fiber: 3.58g

## 56 "OATMEAL COOKIE" BAKED OATMEAL

Prep Time: 10 mins
Cook Time: 45 mins
Total Time: 55 mins
Servings: 4

### *Ingredients*

- 1.5 cups unsweetened applesauce
- 1 large egg
- 1/2 cup brown sugar
- 1/2 Tbsp vanilla extract
- 1/2 Tbsp cinnamon
- 1/4 tsp nutmeg
- 3/4 tsp salt
- 1 tsp baking powder
- 2 Tbsp melted butter
- 1.5 cups milk
- 1/2 cup raisins
- 3 cups old-fashioned rolled oats

### *Instructions*

- Preheat the oven to 375ºF. In a large bowl, whisk together the apple sauce, egg, brown sugar, vanilla, cinnamon, nutmeg, salt, baking powder, and melted butter. Once whisked

smooth, add the milk and whisk until smooth again.
- Add the raisins and dry rolled oats. Stir with a spoon until the mixture is combined. Lightly coat a 9x9 casserole dish (or any 2-3 quart casserole dish) with non-stick spray, then pour the oat mixture into the dish.
- Bake the oatmeal uncovered in the fully preheated oven for 45 minutes. Divide into six portions and serve. Baked oatmeal is good warm or cold and tastes great with cold milk poured over top.

### *Nutrition Info*

Calories: 370.6kcal, Carbohydrates: 65.2g, Protein: 8.58g, Fat: 9.33g, Sodium: 432.12mg, Fiber: 5.48g

# 57 CRISPY HASH BROWNS

Prep Time: 15 mins
Cook Time: 15 mins
Total Time: 30 mins
Servings: (1 cup each)

## *Ingredients*

- 2 large russet potatoes (about 2 lbs.)
- 4 Tbsp cooking oil, or as needed
- Seasoning salt to taste

## *Instructions*

- Peel the potatoes, if desired. Use a large-holed cheese grater or food processor to shred the potatoes. Place the potatoes in a colander and rinse well, or until the water runs clear. Let the potatoes drain.
- Squeeze the potatoes of their excess water by pressing against the side of the colander or squeezing in your fist. Or, place the potatoes in a clean, lint-free dish towel, roll them up, then press to remove excess moisture.
- Heat a large cast iron or non-stick skillet over medium heat. Once hot, add a tablespoon of cooking oil. Tilt the skillet to spread the oil over the surface. Add about 1/3 of the shredded

potatoes or enough to cover the surface of the skillet in a solid, yet thin layer (1/2 inch thick or so). Let the potatoes fry, without disturbing, until deeply golden brown on the bottom (3-5 minutes). Season lightly with seasoning salt.
- Flip the potatoes, and drizzle with additional oil if needed. Let the potatoes cook on the second side without disturbing until golden brown and crispy again. Season lightly on the second side.
- If needed, flip and cook one more time to achieve the ratio of brown to white that you like. Repeat the process until all of the potatoes are cooked. Serve hot.

### Nutrition Info

Calories: 288.35kcal, Carbohydrates: 39.98g, Protein: 4.63g, Fat: 14g, Sodium: 147.5mg, Fiber: 3.18g

# 58 WEEKNIGHT ENCHILADAS

Prep Time: 10 mins
Cook Time: 45 mins
Total Time: 55 mins
Servings: 4 enchiladas each

## *Ingredients*

SAUCE

- 2 Tbsp vegetable or canola oil
- 2 Tbsp chili powder
- 2 Tbsp flour
- 2 cups water
- 3 oz. tomato paste
- ½ tsp cumin
- ½ tsp garlic powder
- ¼ tsp cayenne pepper
- ¾ tsp salt

ENCHILADAS

- 16 small corn tortillas
- 4 cups refried beans
- 8 oz. Pepper Jack, shredded (2 cups)
- 1/2 large avocado, sliced thin
- 1/4 bunch cilantro (or green onions), roughly chopped

*Instructions*

- Begin by making the sauce. In a small sauce pot, combine the chili powder, flour, and oil. Heat over a medium flame, while stirring, for one to two minutes to toast the spices and flour. Whisk in the water, tomato paste, cumin, garlic powder, and cayenne pepper. Allow the mixture to come to a simmer, at which point it will thicken. Once thick enough to coat a spoon, taste and add salt as needed (1/2 to 3/4 tsp). Set the sauce aside.
- Toast the tortillas in a dry skillet over medium flame until they are just flecked with brown on each side. The tortillas should be slightly more firm, but still pliable enough to roll. Stack the tortillas on a clean plate as they come out of the skillet.
- Prepare a casserole dish by coating with non-stick spray, then spread a layer of enchilada sauce over the bottom (1/2 to 1 cup). Preheat the oven to 350 degrees.
- Add about 1/4 cup of refried beans to each tortilla, plus a small pinch of shredded cheese. Roll the tortilla tightly around the beans and cheese, then place seam side down in the casserole dish. Continue until all of the tortillas are filled. Pour another 1/2 to 1 cup enchilada sauce over the rolled enchiladas in the dish,

leaving some of the edges exposed so they can become brown and crispy. Top with the remaining shredded cheese.
- Bake the casserole in the oven for 25-30 minutes or until the sauce is thick and bubbly around the edges and the center is heated through. Top with thin slices of avocado and chopped cilantro leaves (or sliced green onions).

***Nutrition Info***

Calories: 748.4kcal, Carbohydrates: 80.73g, Protein: 33.65g, Fat: 33.18g, Sodium: 1891.68mg, Fiber: 21.28g

# 59 TROPICAL YOGURT PARFAITS

Prep Time: 15 mins
Total Time: 15 mins
Servings: 4

## *Ingredients*

- 1 cup rolled oats
- 1 1/3 cup yogurt
- 2 bananas
- 1 20oz. can pineapple chunks in juice
- 1 mango
- 4 Tbsp shredded coconut

## *Instructions*

- Add 1/4 cup rolled oats to the bottom of four 12oz. mason jars, or another container of comparable size. Add 1/3 cup of yogurt on top of the oats in each jar.
- Slice the bananas, drain the pineapple (the juice can be saved for smoothies), and dice the mango. Divide the sliced bananas, pineapple chunks, and mango between the four jars. Layering the bananas between the yogurt and pineapple will help prevent the banana from browning. Top each jar off with a tablespoon of shredded coconut.

- Refrigerate the jars overnight to allow the oats time to soak and soften. Use a spoon to stir the ingredients in the jar just before eating. Refrigerate the parfaits for up to five days.

### Nutrition Info

Calories: 316.93kcal, Carbohydrates: 62.45g, Protein: 7.68g, Fat: 6.75g, Sodium: 80.38mg, Fiber: 5.75g

## 60 BROILED BALSAMIC VEGETABLES WITH LEMON PARSLEY RICE

Prep Time: 20 mins
Cook Time: 40 mins
Total Time: 1 hr
Servings: to 6 servings

### Ingredients

BALSAMIC MARINADE

- 2 Tbsp olive oil
- 1/4 cup balsamic vinegar
- 2 cloves garlic, minced
- 2 Tbsp brown sugar
- 2 Tbsp soy sauce
- 1 Tbsp Dijon mustard
- Freshly cracked pepper

VEGETABLES

- 8 oz. button mushrooms
- 1 green bell pepper
- 1 zucchini
- 4 oz. grape tomatoes
- 1 yellow or red onion

LEMON PARSLEY RICE

- 1.5 cups long grain white rice
- 2.5 cups water
- 1 clove garlic, minced
- 1/2 tsp salt
- 1/2 bunch fresh parsley
- 2 Tbsp olive oil
- Zest of one lemon

## *Instructions*

- In a small bowl, stir together the ingredients for the balsamic marinade (olive oil, balsamic vinegar, garlic, brown sugar, soy sauce, Dijon, and some freshly cracked pepper).
- Cut the mushrooms, bell pepper, zucchini, and onion into one-inch cubes, or as close to that size as possible. Leave the grape tomatoes whole. Place the vegetables in a gallon-sized zip top bag and pour the marinade over top. Massage the bag to mix the vegetables with the marinade. Let them marinate for 30 minutes at room temperature, flipping the bag occasionally to redistribute the marinade.
- While the vegetables are marinating, begin the rice. Combine the uncooked rice, water, minced garlic, and salt in a medium pot. Place a lid on top and bring the pot up to a boil over high heat. As soon as it reaches a boil, turn the heat down

to low and let the pot simmer for 15 minutes. After 15 minutes, turn the heat off and let it rest for 5 more minutes, then fluff with a fork. Allow the rice to cool slightly.

- While the rice is cooking, prepare the lemon parsley mix. Pull the leaves from about 1/2 bunch of parsley. Finely chop the leaves until they appear minced. Use a zester, microplane, or small-holed cheese grater to remove the zest from one lemon. Combine the minced parsley, about 1/2 Tbsp lemon zest, and olive oil in a small bowl.
- When the rice has cooled just slightly, add the lemon parsley mix and fold gently until the rice is coated in parsley, lemon, and olive oil. Avoid vigorous stirring, as this can make the rice pasty.
- Adjust the oven rack to the second position from the top and preheat the broiler on high. Cover a large baking sheet with parchment. Spread the marinated vegetables out over the surface of the baking sheet. If they do not cover the sheet in a single layer, use two baking sheets to avoid over crowding.
- Broil the vegetables about 6-8 inches from the flame for 10 minutes, or until they achieve a subtle char on the edges. Every broiler is slightly different, so keep a close eye on them and turn the baking sheet as needed. For more even broiling, stir the vegetables half way through.

- Fill each bowl with a scoop of lemon parsley rice and a pile of the broiled balsamic vegetables.

### *Nutrition Info*

Calories: 457.63kcal, Carbohydrates: 74.85g, Protein: 8.5g, Fat: 14.18g, Sodium: 886.65mg, Fiber: 2.95g

# 61 SESAME KALE

Prep Time: 10 mins
Cook Time: 7 mins
Total Time: 17 mins
Servings: 4

## Ingredients

- 1 bunch lacinato (dino) kale
- 1 Tbsp cooking oil
- 2 cloves garlic
- 1 Tbsp soy sauce
- 1 tsp toasted sesame oil
- 1 Tbsp sesame seeds

## Instructions

- Remove the woody stems from the kale leaves either by slicing down each side with a sharp knife, or by pinching the leaf at the base and pulling out toward the tip. Stack the leaves and then slice crosswise into one inch wide strips. Wash the leaves well in a colander with cool running water.
- Mince the of garlic and add it to a large pot with one tablespoon of neutral cooking oil (or your favorite cooking oil). Sauté the garlic for about one minute over medium heat.

- Add the washed kale leaves to the pot. Stir and cook the kale until it is wilted and glossy (about 5 minutes). If you prefer a more tender leaf, cook longer.
- Add the soy sauce, toasted sesame oil, and sesame seeds to the pot. Stir to coat. Taste and adjust the seasoning to your liking. Serve warm.

### *Nutrition Info*

Calories: 67.95kcal, Carbohydrates: 3.43g, Protein: 1.85g, Fat: 5.88g, Sodium: 230.28mg, Fiber: 1.3g

# 62 BLUEBERRY BUTTERMILK COFFEE CAKE

Prep Time: 15 mins
Cook Time: 45 mins
Total Time: 1 hr
Servings: 8

## Ingredients

STREUSEL TOPPING

- 1/4 cup all-purpose flour
- 1/4 cup brown sugar
- 2 Tbsp softened butter
- 1/2 tsp cinnamon

COFFEE CAKE

- 2 cups all-purpose flour
- 1 Tbsp baking powder
- 3/4 tsp baking soda
- 1/4 tsp salt
- 1/2 cup white sugar
- 2 large eggs
- 1 cup buttermilk
- 1/4 cup melted butter
- 1/2 cup blueberries (frozen or fresh)

## Instructions

- Preheat the oven to 350ºF. In a small bowl, combine the ingredients for the streusel topping (flour, brown sugar, softened butter, and cinnamon) until they create a uniform, crumbly topping. Set the topping aside.
- In a large bowl, stir together the flour, baking powder, baking soda, and salt for the coffee cake batter. In a separate bowl, whisk together the white sugar, eggs, buttermilk, and melted butter until smooth. Pour the bowl of wet ingredients into the bowl of dry ingredients, and stir just until a thick, fluffy batter forms (do not over stir).
- Coat an 8x8 inch baking dish (or similar size) with nonstick spray. Spread the batter into the dish. Sprinkle the blueberries over top, then push them down into the batter with your fingers. Sprinkle the streusel topping over the top.
- Bake the coffee cake in the fully preheated 350ºF oven for 40-45 minutes, or until the top is golden brown. Slice into eight pieces, then serve.

### *Nutrition Info*

Calories: 322.61kcal, Carbohydrates: 49.45g, Protein: 6.3g, Fat: 11.3g, Sodium: 447.46mg, Fiber: 1.3g

# 63 BROCCOLI CHEDDAR STUFFED BAKED POTATOES

Prep Time: 10 mins
Cook Time: 1 hr
Total Time: 1 hr 10 mins
Servings: 4

## *Ingredients*

BAKED POTATOES

- 4 russet potatoes (about ¾ lb. each)
- 1 Tbsp olive oil
- Salt

BROCCOLI CHEESE SAUCE

- 1/2 lb frozen broccoli florets
- 3 Tbsp butter
- 3 Tbsp all-purpose flour
- 3 cups whole milk
- 1 tsp salt
- 1/4 tsp garlic powder
- 6 oz. medium cheddar, shredded

## *Instructions*

- Preheat the oven to 400ºF. Take the broccoli out of the freezer and allow it to thaw as the potatoes bake. Once thawed, roughly chop the broccoli into small pieces and then set aside until ready to use.
- Wash the potatoes well, then dry with paper towel or a clean dish towel. Use a fork to prick several holes in the skin of each potato. Pour the olive oil into a small dish, then use your hands to coat each potato in oil. Place the oil coated potatoes on a baking sheet, and season with a pinch of salt. Bake the potatoes for about 60 minutes, or until tender all the way through.
- When there is about 15 minutes left in the baking time for the potatoes, begin to prepare the cheese sauce. Add the butter and flour to a medium sauce pot. Place the pot over a medium flame and whisk the butter and flour together as they melt. Allow the mixture to begin to bubble and foam, whisking continuously. Continue to cook for 2 minutes more to remove the raw flour flavor, but do not let the flour begin to brown.
- Whisk the milk into the butter and flour mixture. Bring the milk up to a simmer, whisking frequently. When it reaches a simmer, it will thicken. Once thick enough to coat a spoon, turn off the heat. Season the white sauce with the salt and garlic powder.

- Begin to whisk the shredded cheddar into the sauce one handful at a time, making sure the cheese is fully melted into the sauce before adding the next handful. Once all of the cheddar has been melted into the sauce, stir in the chopped broccoli.
- When the potatoes are finished baking, carefully slice them open. Use a fork to slightly mash the insides of the potatoes. When ready to serve, place each potato on a plate or in a bowl and ladle the broccoli cheese sauce over each potato. Serve warm.

**Nutrition Info**

Calories: 602.58kcal, Carbohydrates: 56.2g, Protein: 23.35g, Fat: 32.8g, Sodium: 1123.25mg, Fiber: 5.1g

## 64 CHIMICHURRI SAUCE: GOOD ON ANYTHING AND EVERYTHING

Prep Time: 10 mins
Total Time: 10 mins
Servings: 2 Tbsp each

### Ingredients

- 1 cup Italian parsley, packed
- 1/2 cup fresh cilantro, packed
- 1/2 cup olive oil
- 1/4 cup red wine vinegar
- 3 cloves garlic
- 1 tsp dried oregano*
- 1/2 tsp ground cumin
- 1/4 tsp crushed red pepper
- 1/2 tsp salt

### Instructions

- Rinse the parsley and cilantro well to remove any dirt or debris. Shake as much water off the leaves as possible. Pull the parsley and cilantro leaves from their stems, then chop them finely. Mince the garlic.
- Combine the olive oil, red wine vinegar, garlic, oregano, cumin, crushed red pepper, salt,

chopped parsley, and chopped cilantro in a bowl. Stir to combine.
- Use the chimichurri immediately or refrigerate until ready to use.

**Nutrition Info**

Calories: 167.17kcal, Carbohydrates: 1.52g, Protein: 0.48g, Fat: 18.13g, Sodium: 203.6mg, Fiber: 0.55g

## 65 KALE SALAD WITH CAJUN SPICED CHICKPEAS AND BUTTERMILK DRESSING

Prep Time: 20 mins
Cook Time: 5 mins
Total Time: 25 mins
Servings: 4

### Ingredients

BUTTERMILK DRESSING

- 1/2 cup buttermilk
- 1/3 cup mayonnaise
- 1 Tbsp lemon juice
- 1/4 tsp salt (plus more to taste)
- 1/4 tsp garlic powder
- 1/4 tsp dried oregano
- Freshly cracked black pepper

CAJUN SPICED CHICKPEAS*

- 1 15oz. can chickpeas
- 1 Tbsp olive oil
- 1/4 tsp salt
- 1/2 tsp smoked paprika
- 1/4 tsp garlic powder
- 1/8 tsp onion powder
- 1/4 tsp dried oregano

- 1/8 tsp cayenne pepper
- 1/8 tsp dried thyme
- Freshly cracked black pepper

SALAD

- 1 bunch lacinato kale (about 1/2 lb.)
- 1/4 red onion
- 1.5 Tbsp grated Parmesan

### Instructions

- Prepare the dressing first, so the flavors have time to blend. In a medium bowl, whisk together the buttermilk dressing ingredients (buttermilk, mayonnaise, lemon juice, salt, garlic powder, oregano, and about 10-15 cranks of a pepper mill). Taste the dressing and add more salt if desired. Refrigerate the dressing until ready to use.
- Drain the chickpeas in a colander and rinse with cool water. Add the olive oil to a non-stick skillet and place over a medium flame. Add the drained chickpeas along with the salt, smoked paprika, garlic powder, onion powder, oregano, cayenne, thyme, and another 10-15 cranks of a pepper mill. Sauté the chickpeas and spices for about five minutes, or until the chickpeas are slightly toasted. Remove from the heat.

- Remove the stems from the kale, then slice the kale leaves into thin strips (see step by step photos below for more detail). Rinse the kale with cool water and allow the excess water to drain away. Thinly slice the red onion.
- To build the salad, place the washed kale in a large bowl (or four serving bowls), add the spiced chickpeas, a few slices of red onion, and a light dusting of Parmesan (about 1 tsp per serving). Finally, taste the buttermilk dressing after it has had time to refrigerate and adjust the salt if needed. Drizzle the dressing over the salad and then serve.

### *Nutrition Info*

Calories: 341.23kcal, Carbohydrates: 27.68g, Protein: 9.83g, Fat: 22.53g, Sodium: 1042.65mg, Fiber: 8.1g

## 66 SLOW COOKER COCONUT CURRY LENTILS

Prep Time: 30 mins
Cook Time: 4 hrs
Total Time: 4 hrs 30 mins
Servings: 10 cups

### Ingredients

COCONUT CURRY LENTILS

- 1 yellow onion
- 2 cloves garlic
- 2 cups brown lentils
- 1 sweet potato (about 3/4 lb.)
- 2 carrots
- 3 Tbsp curry powder (hot or mild)
- 1/4 tsp ground cloves (optional)
- 1 15oz. can petite diced tomatoes
- 1 15oz. can tomato sauce
- 3 cups vegetable broth*
- 1 14oz. can coconut milk (full fat)

FOR SERVING

- 10 cups cooked rice
- 1/2 red onion
- 1/2 bunch fresh cilantro or green onions

## Instructions

- Dice the onion and mince the garlic. Peel the sweet potato and carrots. Dice the sweet potato (1/4-1/2 inch cubes) and slice the carrots.
- Add the onion, garlic, sweet potato, carrots, lentils, curry powder, cloves, diced tomatoes, tomato sauce, and vegetable broth to the slow cooker. Stir to combine. Place the lid on the slow cooker and cook on high for 4 hours or low for 7-8 hours. Once cooked, the lentils should be tender and most of the liquid should be absorbed.
- Stir the can of coconut milk into the lentils. Taste and adjust the salt or other spices as needed (the amount of salt needed will depend on the type of broth used and the salt content of the canned tomatoes).
- To serve, add 1 cup cooked rice to a bowl followed by 1 cup of the lentil mixture. Top with finely diced red onion and fresh cilantro.

## Nutrition Info

Calories: 430.69kcal, Carbohydrates: 87.67g, Protein: 16.16g, Fat: 2.14g, Sodium: 943.99mg, Fiber: 8.68g

## 67 VEGGIE PACKED FREEZER BREAKFAST SANDWICHES

Prep Time: 1 hr
Cook Time: 30 mins
Total Time: 1 hr 30 mins
Servings: 6

### *Ingredients*

- 6 large eggs
- 1/2 cup milk
- 1/2 tsp salt
- Freshly cracked pepper
- 1/2 lb. frozen cut leaf spinach
- 1/2 12 oz. jar roasted red peppers
- 6 English Muffins
- 6 slices cheese

### *Instructions*

- Preheat the oven to 350ºF. In a large bowl, whisk together the eggs, milk, salt, and pepper.
- Thaw the spinach (I used the microwave), then squeeze out the excess moisture. Take the peppers out of the liquid in the jar, then slice into thin strips. Cut the pepper strips crosswise into smaller pieces. Stir the spinach and peppers into the egg mixture.

- Coat an 8x9 or 8x12 inch casserole dish with nonstick spray. Pour the egg and vegetable mixture into the dish. Bake the eggs for about 30 minutes, or until the center is set and the outer edges are slightly browned. Allow the eggs to cool, then slice into six pieces.
- Build the sandwiches by adding one piece of the baked eggs and one slice of cheese to each English muffin. Wrap each sandwich in plastic wrap or a fold top sandwich bag, then place all the sandwiches in a gallon sized freezer bag. Freeze for up to 2 months.
- To reheat, unwrap the sandwich, place on a microwave safe plate, then microwave on the defrost setting for one minute. Following the defrost, heat on high for 30 seconds at a time until heated through. Or, thaw in the refrigerator over night and simply microwave on high until heated through.

# 68 HOMEMADE PINEAPPLE ORANGE JULIUS

Prep Time: 5 mins
Total Time: 5 mins
Servings: 12 oz.

## Ingredients

- 1/4 cup orange juice concentrate
- 1/2 cup frozen pineapple
- 1/2 tsp vanilla extract
- 1 Tbsp sugar*
- 1 cup whole milk

## Instructions

- Place all the ingredients in a blender and blend until smooth and frothy. Drink immediately.
- For a thicker drink, add a few ice cubes or more frozen pineapple. For a thinner drink, add more milk.

## Nutrition Info

Calories: 340.3kcal, Carbohydrates: 58.3g, Protein: 10.1g, Fat: 8.3g, Sodium: 125.7mg, Fiber: 1.9g

# 69 NO-CHURN MINT CHOCOLATE CHIP ICE CREAM

Prep Time: 8 hrs 30 mins
Total Time: 8 hrs 30 mins
Servings: 6 cups

## Ingredients

- 14 oz can sweetened condensed milk
- 1 1/2 tsp mint extract
- 1/2 tsp vanilla extract
- 1 pint heavy whipping cream
- 1/4 cup mini chocolate chips
- 1/4 cup chocolate syrup

## Instructions

- Chill a 2 quart or larger glass or metal casserole dish or bread pan in the freezer while you prepare the ice cream mixture.
- In a medium bowl, stir together the sweetened condensed milk, mint extract, and vanilla extract.
- In a separate large bowl, whip the heavy whipping cream until stiff peaks form (use a hand mixer or a whisk and some elbow grease). Be sure not to over whip the cream to the point where it breaks down and separates.

- Take a scoop of the whipped cream and fold it into the bowl with the sweetened condensed milk. This will help lighten the thick condensed milk a bit.
- Now take about 1/3 of the sweetened condensed milk and fold it into the bowl of whipped cream. Fold gently until it is incorporated, then add 1/3 more and gently fold the mixture again. Repeat this process until all the sweetened condensed milk is incorporated into the whipped cream and the mixture is smooth.
- Spoon the ice cream mixture into the chilled dish and spread the top smooth. Cover and chill the mixture for two hours. After chilling, drizzle the chocolate syrup over top and add the chocolate chips. Gently fold the syrup and chips into the chilled mixture to create a marbled texture (don't over stir). Return the ice cream to the freezer and freeze until solid (6-8 hours). Scoop and enjoy!

### *Nutrition Info*

Calories: 635.08kcal, Carbohydrates: 65.07g, Protein: 10.27g, Fat: 39.02g, Sodium: 142.63mg, Fiber: 1g

## 70 ULTIMATE SOUTHWEST SCRAMBLED EGGS

Prep Time: 10 mins
Cook Time: 15 mins
Total Time: 25 mins
Servings: 4

### *Ingredients*

- 8 large eggs
- 1/4 cup milk
- salt and pepper
- 1 Tbsp butter
- 1 15oz. can black beans
- 1 4oz. can diced green chiles
- 1/4 cup taco sauce
- 4 oz. pepper jack, shredded
- 2 green onions
- 1 small tomato

### *Instructions*

- Rinse the can of beans in a colander and let drain as you prepare the eggs.
- In a large bowl, combine the eggs, milk, a pinch of salt, and pepper. Whisk until fairly smooth.
- Heat a large skillet over medium-low heat. Once hot, add the butter and let it melt. Spread the butter over the surface of the skillet with a

spatula. Pour the whisked eggs into the skillet and gently fold them with the spatula as they begin to set. Avoid over stirring the eggs.
- When the eggs are bout 75% set (still soft, moist, and fluid around the edges), add the drained beans and chopped green chiles (no need to drain the chiles). Gently fold the beans and chiles into the scrambled eggs. Drizzle taco sauce over the eggs, then top with pepper jack.
- Place a lid on the skillet and let it warm for about 5 more minutes, or until the eggs are fully set and the cheese on top is melted.
- While the eggs are warming through, slice the green onions and dice the tomato. Top the eggs with the fresh tomato and green onion just before serving.

### *Nutrition Info*

Calories: 458.5kcal, Carbohydrates: 33.25g, Protein: 30.75g, Fat: 22.93g, Sodium: 1182.15mg, Fiber: 12.3g

# 71 CHEDDAR GRITS BREAKFAST BOWLS

Prep Time: 10 mins
Cook Time: 20 mins
Total Time: 30 mins
Servings: 4

## *Ingredients*

- 4 cups water
- 1 tsp salt
- 1 cup quick cooking yellow grits
- 2 Tbsp butter
- 1/2 cup whole milk
- 4 oz medium cheddar, grated
- 4 large eggs
- 1 cup salsa
- 4 green onions, sliced
- Freshly cracked pepper

## *Instructions*

- Add the water and salt to a medium sauce pot. Place a lid on top, turn the heat on to high, and bring the water up to a rolling boil. Once boiling, stir in the grits. Turn the heat down to low, replace the lid, and let simmer for 5-7 minutes, or until thickened.*

- Add the butter and milk to the grits and stir until the butter has melted and the grits are smooth. Stir in the grated cheddar, one handful at a time, until fully melted in and smooth. Leave the lid on the pot with the burner turned off to keep the grits warm.
- Cook four eggs using your favorite method (fried, scrambled, soft boiled, etc.). Slice the green onions.
- To build the bowls, place one cup of the cheddar grits in a bowl, top with one egg, 1/4 cup salsa, some freshly cracked pepper, and a sprinkle of sliced green onions.

### *Nutrition Info*

Calories: 427.23kcal, Carbohydrates: 38.83g, Protein: 17.4g, Fat: 21.4g, Sodium: 1420.95mg, Fiber: 3.08g

## 72 CHIPOTLE PORTOBELLO OVEN FAJITAS

Prep Time: 15 mins
Cook Time: 40 mins
Total Time: 55 mins
Servings: 4 (two fajitas each)

### *Ingredients*

FAJITA SPICE MIX

- 1 Tbsp chili powder*
- 1/2 tsp chipotle powder
- 1/2 tsp onion powder
- 1 tsp cumin
- 1/2 tsp garlic powder
- 1 tsp sugar**
- 1/2 tsp salt

FAJITAS

- 2 portobello mushroom caps
- 2 bell peppers (any color)
- 2 yellow onions
- 3 Tbsp olive oil
- 8 small (6 inch) flour tortillas
- 1 avocado
- Handful cilantro (optional)
- 1 fresh lime

## Instructions

- Preheat the oven to 400ºF. In a small bowl, stir together all the ingredients for the fajita spice mix
- Slice the portobellos, bell peppers, and onions into 1/4 inch wide strips. Place the sliced vegetables in a large 9x13 inch casserole dish or on a large baking sheet. Drizzle the olive oil over the vegetables then sprinkle the fajita spice mix over top. Use your hands to toss the vegetables until everything is well coated in oil and spices.
- Roast the vegetables in the fully preheated oven for 40 minutes, or until the vegetables are slightly wilted and the edges have a nice brown color. Stir the vegetables half way through the roasting time to make sure everything gets even exposure to the hot air.
- After removing the vegetables from the oven, squeeze fresh lime juice over top. Sprinkle chopped cilantro over the vegetables. To serve the fajitas, scoop a small amount of the roasted vegetables into each tortilla and add a slice of avocado.

## Nutrition Info

Calories: 517.5kcal, Carbohydrates: 62.55g, Protein: 11.23g, Fat: 27.08g, Sodium: 1087.45mg, Fiber: 6.9g

## 73 TOMATO HERB RICE WITH WHITE BEANS AND SPINACH

Prep Time: 10 mins
Cook Time: 45 mins
Total Time: 55 mins
Servings: 8 cups total/1.33 cups each

### *Ingredients*

- 2 Tbsp olive oil
- 2 cloves garlic
- 1/2 tsp dried oregano
- 1/2 tsp dried basil
- 1/4 tsp dried thyme
- 1/4 tsp dried rosemary
- 1 pinch crushed red pepper
- Freshly cracked black pepper
- 3 oz. tomato paste (about 1/4 cup)
- 1/2 tsp brown sugar
- 1/4 tsp salt
- 1 yellow onion
- 1 15oz. can fire roasted diced tomatoes
- 1 15oz. can cannellini beans
- 1/4 lb. frozen chopped spinach
- 1 cup uncooked long grain white rice
- 1.5 cups vegetable broth*

### *Instructions*

- Place the spinach in a bowl and allow it to thaw slightly as you prepare the beginning of the recipe.
- Dice the onion and mince the garlic. Set the onion aside. Add the olive oil, minced garlic, oregano, basil, thyme, rosemary, a pinch of crushed red pepper, and a little freshly cracked black pepper (about 10 cranks of a pepper mill) to a heavy bottomed pot or deep skillet. Sauté the garlic and spices over medium-low heat for about one minute.
- Add the tomato paste and brown sugar to the pot and continue to sauté for 2-3 minutes, or until the tomato paste takes on a deep burgundy color. Add the onion and salt and continue to sauté for a few minutes more, or until the onions become soft and transparent.
- Meanwhile, drain and rinse the cannellini beans in a colander. Add the diced tomatoes (with juices), cannellini beans, spinach, and uncooked rice to the pot. Pour in the vegetable broth and stir briefly to combine the ingredients.
- Place a lid on the pot and turn the heat up to medium-high. Allow the contents to come up to a boil. Once it reaches a boil, turn the heat down to the lowest setting that allows the liquid to maintain a simmer. Let the pot simmer for 15-20 minutes, or until most of the liquid is

absorbed (there may still be some around the edges. Turn the heat off and let the pot rest, undisturbed, for 10 additional minutes.
- Finally, fluff the contents of the pot with a fork, making sure to not stir vigorously. Serve immediately.

## *Nutrition Info*

Calories: 316kcal, Carbohydrates: 55.77g, Protein: 11.75g, Fat: 5.6g, Sodium: 766.47mg, Fiber: 7.37g

# 74 PRESSURE COOKER SPLIT PEA SOUP

Prep Time: 10 mins
Cook Time: 45 mins
Total Time: 55 mins
Servings: 9 cups total

## *Ingredients*

- 1 yellow onion
- 3 carrots
- 3 ribs celery
- 2 cloves garlic
- 1 lb split peas
- 2 Tbsp coconut oil
- 1 bay leaf
- 1/2 Tbsp smoked paprika
- 1/4 tsp thyme
- Freshly cracked pepper
- 6 cups vegetable broth

## *Instructions*

- Dice the onion, slice the carrots and celery, and mince the garlic. Place the onion, carrots, celery, and garlic in the pressure cooker along with all the remaining ingredients.
- Secure the lid on the pressure cooker, close the steam valve, and set the cooker to high pressure

for 15 minutes (Instant Pot: Manual function, set time to 15 minutes). After 15 minutes of high pressure, allow the cooker to release pressure naturally. (Total cook time with coming up to pressure, cooking, and natural pressure release is approximately 45 minutes.)
- Once the cooker returns to normal pressure, open the steam valve, open the lid, and stir the soup. Taste and adjust the salt or other seasonings as needed. Serve hot with crusty bread for dipping.

### Nutrition Info

Calories: 352.37kcal, Carbohydrates: 55.87g, Protein: 18.2g, Fat: 7.62g, Sodium: 883.45mg, Fiber: 18.52g

# 75 SOUTHWEST SPAGHETTI SqUASH BOWLS

Prep Time: 15 mins
Cook Time: 2 mins
Total Time: 17 mins
Servings: 4

## Ingredients

- 4 cups cooked spaghetti squash
- 1/2 Tbsp chili powder*
- Salt to taste
- 1 15oz. can black beans
- 1 cup salsa
- 4 oz. Monterey jack cheese
- 2 green onions

## Instructions

- Place the cooked spaghetti squash in a bowl. Sprinkle the chili powder and a pinch of salt over the spaghetti squash. Toss the spaghetti squash in the seasoning until evenly covered. Taste and adjust the salt if needed.
- Drain the black beans, shred the cheese, and slice the green onions. Divide the spaghetti squash between four bowls, then add 1/3 cup beans and 1/4 cup salsa to each bowl. Top each bowl with shredded cheese and a few sliced

green onions. Refrigerate until ready to eat. Reheat in the microwave just before serving (one minute on high, stir, then add more time in 30 second intervals until heated through).

## *Nutrition Info*

Calories: 260.55kcal, Carbohydrates: 29.05g, Protein: 14.18g, Fat: 9.9g, Sodium: 827.1mg, Fiber: 11.08g

# 76 FREEZER READY MINI PIZZAS

Prep Time: 8 hrs
Cook Time: 15 mins
Total Time: 8 hrs 15 mins
Servings: 12 pizzas

## *Ingredients*

- 6 English Muffins
- 3/4 cup pizza sauce
- 1.5 cups shredded mozzarella
- Salad Bar Vegetables

## *Instructions*

- Line two small baking sheets with foil or parchment paper (or do one sheet at a time, preparing the second batch the second day). Open the English muffins and line them up on the baking sheets with cut sides facing up.
- Spread about 1 Tbsp pizza sauce over the surface of each muffin, then top with about 2 Tbsp shredded mozzarella.
- Chop the salad bar vegetables into very small pieces, then divide them evenly among the pizzas. Press down lightly on top of each pizza to help compact the toppings and keep them in place as they freeze. Cover the baking sheets

with plastic wrap and freeze for about 8 hours, or until the pizzas are solid.
- Once the pizzas are frozen solid, carefully transfer them to a gallon sized freezer bag for long term storage (you may need two bags). For the best results, the pizzas should be cooked and eaten within 3 months.
- To bake the pizzas, take out the number you wish to bake, place them on a baking sheet, and let them partially thaw as you preheat the oven to 400ºF (about 7 minutes). Once the oven is fully preheated, bake the pizzas for about 15 minutes, or until the edges are golden brown and the cheese is melted. Baking time will vary depending on your oven and the amount of toppings on the pizzas.

### *Nutrition Info*

Calories: 108.38kcal, Carbohydrates: 15.28g, Protein: 5.48g, Fat: 3.3g, Sodium: 254.68mg, Fiber: 1.33g

# 77 PURPLE POWER BOWLS

Prep Time: 30 mins
Total Time: 30 mins
Servings: 4 bowls

## *Ingredients*

LEMON TAHINI DRESSING (optional)

- 1/3 cup tahini
- 1/3 cup water
- 1/4 cup lemon juice
- 1 clove garlic, crushed
- 1/2 tsp ground cumin
- 1/4 tsp cayenne pepper
- 1/2 tsp salt

SALAD

- 2.5 cups cooked rice or other grain
- 1 15oz. can chickpeas
- 4 oz. baby greens
- 2-3 small beets (2/3 lb.)
- 2 zucchini (1 lb.)
- 3 carrots (3/4 lb.)
- 1 small red cabbage (2 lb.)
- 1 avocado
- 1/2 bunch green onion

- 1/2 cup pepitas

## *Instructions*

- Prepare the dressing by placing all the ingredients in a blender and puréeing until smooth. If you don't have a blender, mince the garlic, then whisk the ingredients together in a bowl. Refrigerate the dressing until ready to use.
- Cool the cooked rice, if needed. Drain the can of chickpeas. Wash the beets, zucchini, and carrots well. Use a food processor or large-holed cheese grater to shred the beets, zucchini, and carrots. Remove any wilted leaves from the cabbage, then cut into quarters, and remove the core. Shred the cabbage using a food processor, or slice thinly with a knife. Slice the avocado and green onion.
- To build the bowls, place about 1/2 cup of the cooked rice in a bowl along with about 1/4 cup of chickpeas. Add a handful of baby greens, shredded beets, zucchini, carrots, and cabbage. Top with a few slices of avocado and a sprinkle of pepitas and sliced onion. Finally, drizzle the lemon tahini dressing liberally over the bowl, then eat.

## 78 CREAMY LEMON DILL GREEK PASTA SALAD

Prep Time: 15 mins
Cook Time: 15 mins
Total Time: 30 mins
Servings: 6 (about 1.5 cups each)

### Ingredients

CREAMY LEMON DILL DRESSING

- 1 5oz. container plain Greek yogurt
- 1/4 cup mayonnaise
- 1 clove garlic, minced
- 1 fresh lemon
- 1/4 tsp salt
- 1/4 tsp dried dill
- Freshly cracked black pepper

PASTA SALAD

- 1 lb. penne
- 1 cup grape tomatoes
- 1 cucumber (about 2 cups chopped)
- 1 15oz. can quartered artichoke hearts
- 1/4 red onion
- 2 oz. feta

## Instructions

- Prepare the dressing first so the flavors have time to blend. Use a zester or small-holed cheese grater to remove the zest from the lemon. In a small bowl, stir together the Greek yogurt, mayonnaise, garlic, 1 Tbsp of the lemon juice, 1/2 tsp of the lemon zest, salt, dill, and some freshly cracked pepper (about 10-15 cranks of a pepper mill). Refrigerate the dressing until ready to use.
- Cook the pasta, in lightly salted water, according to the package directions. Drain the pasta and rinse briefly with cool water to bring the temperature down. Let the pasta drain until it's slightly dry and tacky on the surface.
- While the pasta is cooking, slice the cucumber, then cut the slices into quarter rounds. Slice the grape tomatoes in half. Finely dice the red onion. Drain the artichoke hearts, then roughly chop them. Crumble the feta cheese.
- Once the pasta is cooled and drained, Place it in a large bowl and combine with the cucumber, tomatoes, red onion, artichoke hearts, feta, and creamy lemon dill dressing. Stir to coat. Serve immediately or refrigerate until ready to eat.

## Nutrition Info

Calories: 152.4kcal, Carbohydrates: 66.55g, Protein: 15.25g, Fat: 12g, Sodium: 540.8mg, Fiber: 6.53g

# 79 PARSLEY SCALLION HUMMUS PASTA

Prep Time: 15 mins
Cook Time: 15 mins
Total Time: 30 mins
Servings: 4

## *Ingredients*

- 1 15oz. can chickpeas
- 1/4 cup olive oil
- 1 fresh lemon, or 1/4 cup juice
- 1/4 cup tahini
- 1 clove garlic, or 1/4 tsp garlic powder
- 1/4 tsp ground cumin
- 1/2 tsp salt
- 2 scallions (green onions)
- 1/4 bunch fresh parsley
- 8 oz. pasta

## *Instructions*

- Drain the chickpeas and add them to a food processor along with the olive oil, juice from the lemon (about 1/4 cup), tahini, garlic, cumin, and salt. Pulse the ingredients, adding a small amount of water if needed to keep it moving, until the hummus is smooth.

- Slice the scallions (both white and green ends) and pull the parsley leaves from the stems. Add the green onion and parsley to the hummus in the food processor and process again until only small flecks of green remain. Taste the hummus and adjust the salt, lemon, or garlic if needed.
- Cook 8oz. of your favorite pasta according to the package directions. Reserve one cup of the starchy cooking water, then drain the cooked pasta in a colander. Return the drained pasta to the pot with the heat turned off. Add about 3/4 of the hummus to the pasta and stir until the pasta is evenly coated (add more hummus if needed). Add the reserved pasta water as needed to keep the mixture smooth and saucy. Serve immediately.

### *Nutrition Info*

Calories: 583.28kcal, Carbohydrates: 70.98g, Protein: 19.93g, Fat: 25.4g, Sodium: 649.88mg, Fiber: 11.9g

# 80 CUMIN RICE

Prep Time: 2 mins
Cook Time: 35 mins
Total Time: 37 mins
Servings: 6 1 cup each

## *Ingredients*

- 1 Tbsp butter
- 2 tsp cumin seeds
- 1.5 cups long grain jasmine rice
- 1 clove garlic
- 1/2 tsp salt
- 3 cups water

## *Instructions*

- Add the butter and cumin seeds to a medium sauce pot. Sauté the cumin seeds in the butter over medium-low heat for 1-2 minutes, or just until the butter starts to turn golden brown. Do not let the butter burn.
- Add the uncooked rice to the pot and continue to stir and cook for 2-3 minutes more to toast the rice.
- Mince the garlic and add it to the pot along with the salt and water, and stir to combine. Place a

lid on the pot, turn the heat up to high, and let the liquid come up to a boil.
- Once it reaches a boil, turn the heat down to low and let it simmer (with lid) for 15 minutes. After 15 minutes, turn off the heat and let it sit undisturbed for 10 more minutes before lifting the lid.
- After resting for 10 minutes, remove the lid, fluff with a fork, and serve.

### Nutrition Info

Calories: 188.8kcal, Carbohydrates: 37.48g, Protein: 3.47g, Fat: 2.28g, Sodium: 215.25mg, Fiber: 0.68g

# 81 STRAWBERRY ROSÉ SLUSH

Prep Time: 5 mins
Total Time: 5 mins
Servings: 1

## Ingredients

- 1/4 lb frozen strawberries (unsweetened)
- 1 cup Rosé
- 1 Tbsp powdered sugar

## Instructions

- Add the frozen strawberries, powdered sugar, and rosé to a blender. Blend until the drink is thick and smooth.
- If the drink is too thick to blend properly, add a splash more of rosé. If the drink is too thin, add a couple extra frozen strawberries or a few ice cubes and blend again.

## Nutrition Info

Calories: 251.3kcal, Carbohydrates: 22.3g, Protein: 1.1g, Fat: 0.1g, Sodium: 13.5mg, Fiber: 1.2g

# 82 MARINATED LENTIL SALAD

Prep Time: 10 mins
Cook Time: 20 mins
Total Time: 30 mins
Servings: 6, 1 cup each

## Ingredients

LEMON GARLIC DRESSING

- 1 lemon
- 1/4 cup olive oil
- 2 cloves garlic, minced
- 1/2 Tbsp dried oregano
- 1/2 tsp salt
- Freshly Cracked Pepper

SALAD

- 1 cup dry brown lentils
- 1/2 bunch parsley
- 1 pint grape tomatoes
- 1/4 small red onion
- 2 oz feta, crumbled

## Instructions

- Cook the lentils according to the package directions. For most brown lentils, bring 3 cups of water to boil in a pot, add the lentils, then continue to boil for 20 minutes, or until the lentils are tender. Drain the lentils in a colander and rinse briefly with cool water until they are cooled.
- While the lentils are cooking, prepare the lemon garlic dressing. Use a microplane, zester, or small-holed cheese grater to remove about 1 Tbsp of the lemon's zest (the thin, yellow, outer layer of the peel). Set the zest aside. Juice the lemon and measure 1/4 cup of the juice to use for the dressing. In a small bowl, whisk together the lemon juice, olive oil, minced garlic, oregano, salt, and some freshly cracked pepper. Set the dressing aside.
- Rinse the parsley well, shake off as much water as possible, then pull the leaves from the stems. Roughly chop the parsley leaves. Cut the grape tomatoes in half. Finely dice the red onion.
- When the lentils are cooked, cooled, and well drained, transfer them to a large bowl. Add the chopped parsley, tomatoes, red onion, crumbled feta, lemon zest, and the prepared dressing. Stir to combine the ingredients and coat everything in dressing.

- Serve immediately, or refrigerate until ready to eat. Always stir the salad just before serving to redistribute the dressing and flavors.

**Nutrition Info**

Calories: 238.67kcal, Carbohydrates: 25.93g, Protein: 10.03g, Fat: 11.78g, Sodium: 352.02mg, Fiber: 5.27g

## 83 WARM CORN AND AVOCADO SALAD

Prep Time: 10 mins
Cook Time: 7 mins
Total Time: 17 mins
Servings: (1 cup each)

### Ingredients

- 2 Tbsp cooking oil
- 1 lb. frozen corn kernels, thawed
- Salt and Pepper to taste
- 1/4 tsp cumin
- 1/4 red onion
- 1 avocado
- 1/4 bunch cilantro
- 1 lime

### Instructions

- Make sure to let the corn thaw completely. Heat the cooking oil in a large skillet over medium-high heat. When the oil is very hot and shimmering, add the thawed corn and sauté until the corn becomes golden brown and blistered. Remove the corn from the skillet and place it in a large bowl, season with a pinch of salt, pepper, and 1/4 tsp cumin. Allow the corn to cool slightly.

- While the corn is cooling, prepare the remaining vegetables. Finely dice the red onion, roughly chop the cilantro, and cube the avocado. Add the onion, cilantro, and avocado to the bowl with the corn. Stir briefly.
- Squeeze the juice from half the lime over the salad, stir, and taste. Adjust the salt and lime juice as needed. Serve immediately, or refrigerate until ready to eat.

**Nutrition Info**

Calories: 251.43kcal, Carbohydrates: 30.8g, Protein: 4.78g, Fat: 15.3g, Sodium: 218.05mg, Fiber: 7.5g

# 84 PICKLED RED ONIONS

Prep Time: 10 mins
Cook Time: 5 mins
Total Time: 15 mins

## *Ingredients*

- 1.5 cups sliced red onion
- 1 clove garlic
- 3 Tbsp white sugar
- 1.5 Tbsp salt
- 1/2 tsp peppercorns
- 1 cup white vinegar

## *Instructions*

- Thinly slice the red onion and peel the garlic. Place the onion and garlic in a large glass or ceramic bowl.
- Add the sugar, salt, and peppercorns to a small sauce pot. Add the vinegar and stir until the sugar and salt are dissolved. Place a lid on the pot and bring the mixture up to a boil over medium-high heat.
- Once boiling, pour the vinegar over the sliced onion and garlic*. Press the onion down so all the pieces are submerged, then let the mixture cool to room temperature.

- Once cool, use the onions immediately or transfer the onions and all the brine to a lidded non-reactive container (glass, ceramic, or plastic) for storage in the refrigerator. The onions can be stored in the refrigerator for 3-4 weeks.

**Nutrition Info**

Calories: 214.6kcal, Carbohydrates: 53.4g, Protein: 2.1g, Fat: 0.3g, Sodium: 3547.8mg, Fiber: 3.5g

# 85 HARISSA ROASTED VEGETABLES

Prep Time: 15 mins
Cook Time: 40 mins
Total Time: 55 mins
Servings: 6, 1 cup each

## *Ingredients*

HARISSA MARINADE

- 1/4 cup harissa (paste)
- 2 Tbsp olive oil
- 1/2 Tbsp honey
- 1/2 tsp salt
- 1 Tbsp lemon juice

VEGETABLE MEDLEY

- 6 small red potatoes (1-1.5 lbs.)
- 1 broccoli crown
- 3 carrots
- 1 small red onion
- Handful chopped fresh cilantro

## *Instructions*

- Preheat the oven to 400ºF. Prepare a large baking sheet by lightly spritzing with non-stick spray or covering with foil.
- In a small dish, stir together the harissa, olive oil, honey, salt, and lemon juice. Set the marinade aside.
- Wash the potatoes well and cut into one-inch cubes. Wash and peel the carrots, then slice into one-inch sections. Cut the broccoli into florets, and chop the onion into large sections. Place the potatoes, carrots, broccoli, and onion on the prepared baking sheet.
- Pour the harissa marinade over the vegetables and use your hands to toss the vegetables until they are evenly coated in the marinade.
- Roast the vegetables in the preheated oven for 30 minutes, stir, and then continue roasting for another 10 minutes, or until the vegetables are tender and the edges have achieved a nice deep brown color. Top with chopped cilantro just before serving.

**Nutrition Info**

Calories: 184.77kcal, Carbohydrates: 28.02g, Protein: 3.98g, Fat: 7.52g, Sodium: 258.07mg, Fiber: 4.33g

# 86 CHEESY SCALLION STUFFED JALAPEÑOS

Prep Time: 15 mins
Cook Time: 22 mins
Total Time: 37 mins
Servings: 24 pieces (4 per serving)

## *Ingredients*

- 4 oz. cream cheese
- 4 oz. Monterey jack, shredded
- 1/4 cup sour cream
- 3 scallions (green onions), sliced
- 1 clove garlic, minced
- 1/4 cup chopped cilantro leaves
- 1/2 tsp chili powder
- 1/8 tsp salt
- 12 jalapeños
- 1 Tbsp cooking oil

## *Instructions*

- Preheat the oven to 375ºF and line a baking sheet with parchment. In a medium bowl, stir together the cream cheese, Monterey jack, sour cream, scallions, garlic, cilantro, chili powder, and salt.
- Carefully slice each jalapeño down the center, lengthwise. Use a spoon to scrape out the ribs

and seeds. Dip your fingers in the cooking oil and spread the oil over the outer surface of the peppers.
- Spoon about 1 Tbsp of the filling into each hallowed jalapeño half. Arrange the peppers on the prepared baking sheet in a single layer (use two baking sheets if necessary).
- Bake the peppers in the preheated oven for 18-22 minutes, or until the peppers have softened and the cheese on top is slightly browned. Serve hot.

**Nutrition Info**

Calories: 187.42kcal, Carbohydrates: 4.3g, Protein: 6.48g, Fat: 16.53g, Sodium: 233.37mg, Fiber: 1.1g

# 87 TOMATO HERB RICE WITH WHITE BEANS AND SPINACH

Prep Time: 10 mins
Cook Time: 45 mins
Total Time: 55 mins
Servings: 8 cups total/1.33 cups each

## Ingredients

- 2 Tbsp olive oil
- 2 cloves garlic
- 1/2 tsp dried oregano
- 1/2 tsp dried basil
- 1/4 tsp dried thyme
- 1/4 tsp dried rosemary
- 1 pinch crushed red pepper
- Freshly cracked black pepper
- 3 oz. tomato paste (about 1/4 cup)
- 1/2 tsp brown sugar
- 1/4 tsp salt
- 1 yellow onion
- 1 15oz. can fire roasted diced tomatoes
- 1 15oz. can cannellini beans
- 1/4 lb. frozen chopped spinach
- 1 cup uncooked long grain white rice
- 1.5 cups vegetable broth

## Instructions

- Place the spinach in a bowl and allow it to thaw slightly as you prepare the beginning of the recipe.
- Dice the onion and mince the garlic. Set the onion aside. Add the olive oil, minced garlic, oregano, basil, thyme, rosemary, a pinch of crushed red pepper, and a little freshly cracked black pepper (about 10 cranks of a pepper mill) to a heavy bottomed pot or deep skillet. Sauté the garlic and spices over medium-low heat for about one minute.
- Add the tomato paste and brown sugar to the pot and continue to sauté for 2-3 minutes, or until the tomato paste takes on a deep burgundy color. Add the onion and salt and continue to sauté for a few minutes more, or until the onions become soft and transparent.
- Meanwhile, drain and rinse the cannellini beans in a colander. Add the diced tomatoes (with juices), cannellini beans, spinach, and uncooked rice to the pot. Pour in the vegetable broth and stir briefly to combine the ingredients.
- Place a lid on the pot and turn the heat up to medium-high. Allow the contents to come up to a boil. Once it reaches a boil, turn the heat down to the lowest setting that allows the liquid to maintain a simmer. Let the pot simmer for 15-20 minutes, or until most of the liquid is

absorbed (there may still be some around the edges. Turn the heat off and let the pot rest, undisturbed, for 10 additional minutes.
- Finally, fluff the contents of the pot with a fork, making sure to not stir vigorously. Serve immediately.

### *Nutrition Info*

Calories: 316kcal, Carbohydrates: 55.77g, Protein: 11.75g, Fat: 5.6g, Sodium: 766.47mg, Fiber: 7.37g

# 88 SMOKY WHITE BEAN SHAKSHUKA

Prep Time: 5 mins
Cook Time: 25 mins
Total Time: 30 mins
Servings: 4

## *Ingredients*

- 2 Tbsp olive oil
- 4 cloves garlic
- 1 yellow onion
- 1 28oz. can whole peeled tomatoes
- 1/2 Tbsp smoked paprika
- 1 tsp ground cumin
- 1/2 tsp dried oregano
- 1/8 tsp crushed red pepper
- Freshly cracked black pepper
- 1/4 tsp salt, or to taste
- 1 15oz. can cannellini beans
- 4 large eggs
- 1 handful fresh parsley, chopped
- 2 oz. feta, crumbled

## *Instructions*

- Mince the garlic and finely dice the onion. Cook both in a large deep skillet with olive oil over

- medium heat until the onions are soft and transparent (about 5 minutes).
- Add the canned tomatoes and their juices, crushing the tomatoes with your hands as you add them to the skillet. Add the smoked paprika, cumin, oregano, red pepper flakes, and some freshly cracked pepper as well. Stir to combine.
- Allow the sauce to come to a simmer. Let the sauce simmer, stirring occasionally, for 5-7 minutes, or until it has thickened slightly. Add 1/4 tsp salt, then taste the sauce and adjust the salt or other spices to your liking.
- Drain the white beans, add them to the skillet, then stir to combine. Allow the skillet to return to a simmer. Simmer for 2-3 minutes more.
- Crack four eggs into the skillet, then place a lid on top and let them simmer for 5 minutes, or until the whites are set but the yolks are still soft. Top the skillet with the crumbled feta and chopped parsley.

### *Nutrition Info*

Calories: 380.63kcal, Carbohydrates: 47.2g, Protein: 20.23g, Fat: 12.53g, Sodium: 716.38mg, Fiber: 10.43g

# 89 BROCCOLI SALAD WITH HONEY YOGURT DRESSING

Prep Time: 30 mins
Total Time: 30 mins
Servings: 4 (about 6 cups total)

## Ingredients

HONEY YOGURT DRESSING

- 1/2 cup plain Greek yogurt (2%)
- 1/4 cup light mayonnaise
- 1 Tbsp apple cider vinegar
- 1 Tbsp honey
- 1/4 tsp salt
- Freshly cracked pepper to taste

SALAD

- 4 cups broccoli florets (about 2 crowns)
- 1/4 red onion
- 1 carrot
- 1/3 cup dried cranberries
- 1/4 cup raw sunflower seeds

## Instructions

- Prepare the dressing by stirring together the yogurt, mayonnaise, vinegar, honey, salt, and some freshly cracked pepper (about 10-15 cranks of a pepper mill). Set the dressing aside.
- Cut the broccoli into very small florets. Place the florets in a colander and rinse with cool water. Let the broccoli drain while you prepare the rest of the salad ingredients.
- Peel the carrot, then use a large-holed cheese grater to shred the carrot. Slice the red onion into paper thin strips.
- Add the rinsed and well drained broccoli to a large bowl, along with the shredded carrot, sliced red onion, cranberries, and sunflower seeds. Pour the prepared dressing over top, then stir until everything is coated in dressing. Let the salad marinate for 10-15 minutes before serving. Give the salad a brief stir just before serving to redistribute the dressing.

### Nutrition Info

Calories: 205.28kcal, Carbohydrates: 25.6g, Protein: 7.15g, Fat: 9.95g, Sodium: 368.2mg, Fiber: 4.23g

## 90 ULTIMATE PORTOBELLO MUSHROOM PIZZA

Prep Time: 15 mins
Cook Time: 10 mins
Total Time: 25 mins
Servings: 3, 2 slices each

### *Ingredients*

(Not) Sun Dried Tomato Sauce

- 1/4 cup olive oil
- 1 clove garlic, minced
- 1/2 tsp dried oregano
- 1/2 tsp dried basil
- 1/4 tsp dried thyme
- 1/4 tsp dried rosemary
- 1 pinch crushed red pepper
- Freshly cracked black pepper
- 1/2 tsp salt
- 3 oz. tomato paste
- 1/2 tsp honey

Pizza

- 1 large pizza dough
- 1 Tbsp olive oil
- 1 portobello mushroom cap

- Salt and pepper
- 4 oz. shredded mozzarella
- 2 oz. feta, crumbled
- Handful chopped parsley (optional)

## *Instructions*

- Make the (not) Sun Dried Tomato Sauce first. Add the olive oil, garlic, basil, oregano, thyme, rosemary, crushed red pepper, salt, and some freshly cracked pepper to a small skillet. Stir and heat the mixture over low heat for about 3 minutes. It's okay if it sizzles slightly, but you don't want it to get hot enough that the herbs burn.
- Add the tomato paste and honey. Allow it to heat through as you stir. It will not form a smooth sauce. Continue to stir and heat over low for about 5 minutes or until you notice the tomato paste has darkened slightly. Remove the sauce from the heat, then set aside.
- Gently wash any dirt or debris off the portobello mushroom. Cut the mushroom in half, then into thin strips. Add the sliced mushroom to a large skillet with 1 Tbsp olive oil and a pinch of salt and pepper. Cook over medium heat while stirring until the mushroom slices have softened and turned dark brown (3-5 minutes). Set the cooked mushrooms aside.

- Adjust your oven's rack to the highest position and preheat the oven to 500ºF. Stretch the pizza dough out to fit the pizza pan. Spread the
- (Not) Sun Dried Tomato Sauce over the surface of the dough and use any extra oil to brush the crust.
- Sprinkle the mozzarella over the tomato sauce, then add the cooked mushroom pieces and crumbled feta.
- Bake the pizza for 7-10 minutes in the fully preheated oven, or until the cheese is bubbly and slightly browned on top. Finish the baked pizza with a little chopped fresh parsley. Cut the pizza into 6 or 8 pieces and serve.

### Nutrition Info

Calories: 698.17kcal, Carbohydrates: 75.73g, Protein: 23.37g, Fat: 36g, Sodium: 1771.87mg, Fiber: 4.33g

# 91 PEANUT BUTTER AND JELLY BARS

Prep Time: 20 mins
Cook Time: 40 mins
Total Time: 1 hr
Servings: 12 pieces

## *Ingredients*

- 1 1/4 cup all-purpose flour
- 1 cup rolled oats
- 1/4 tsp baking soda
- 1/2 cup salted butter, room temperature
- 1/2 cup brown sugar
- 1 extra large egg
- 1/2 cup natural peanut butter
- 1/2 tsp vanilla extract
- 3/4 cup jam or jelly
- 1/4 cup peanuts

## *Instructions*

- Preheat the oven to 350ºF. Line an 8x8 inch baking dish with parchment or foil.
- In a medium bowl, stir together the flour, oats, and baking soda.
- Using a mixer, cream together the butter and sugar until soft and smooth. Add the egg, peanut butter, and vanilla. Mix until smooth again.

- Pour the flour and oat mixture into the bowl with the peanut butter mixture. Use a spoon to stir until everything is evenly combined and a thick cookie dough forms.
- Press 3/4 of the cookie dough into the bottom of the prepared baking dish in an even layer. Make sure there are no holes or gaps and the dough is compact. Spread the jam evenly over the surface of the cookie dough. Drop the remaining cookie dough over top of the jam in small pieces or crumbles. Sprinkle the peanuts over the top and press them down gently into the jam and dough crumbles. The crumbles and peanuts will not cover the jam in a solid layer.
- Cook the peanut butter and jelly bars for 35-40 minutes, or until the top is golden brown. Let the bars cool slightly, then use the parchment to lift the bars out of the dish. Cut the bars into 12 pieces and enjoy.

### Nutrition Info

Calories: 311.63kcal, Carbohydrates: 39.85g, Protein: 6.28g, Fat: 15.02g, Sodium: 205.86mg, Fiber: 2.36g

# 92 SIMPLE HOMEMADE CRANBERRY SAUCE

Prep Time: 5 mins
Cook Time: 15 mins
Total Time: 20 mins
Servings: 6

## *Ingredients*

- 12 oz bag fresh cranberries
- 1 small orange
- 1/2 cup sugar

## *Instructions*

- Add 1/2 cup sugar and 1 cup water to a medium sauce pot. Stir to combine. Place the pot over medium heat and bring the liquid to a boil.
- While the liquid in the pot is heating, rinse the cranberries. Once the water and sugar are boiling, add the cleaned cranberries and place lid on top. Allow the liquid to come back up to a boil, at which point the cranberries will begin to pop.
- Once all the cranberries have popped, remove the lid, give it a stir, and turn the heat down to medium low. Let the pot continue to simmer over medium-low heat for 5-7 minutes, or until the cranberries have completely broken down.

- While the cranberries simmer, remove the zest from the orange using a microplane, zester, or small-holed cheese grater. Cut the orange in half and squeeze the juice into a bowl (about 1/2 cup juice).
- Once the cranberries have broken down, stir the orange juice into the sauce. Remove the pot from the heat, then stir in about 1 tsp of the orange zest. Allow the sauce to cool slightly, then serve.

### Nutrition Info

Calories: 53.58kcal, Carbohydrates: 14g, Protein: 0.42g, Fat: 0.08g, Sodium: 1.13mg, Fiber: 2.42g

## 93 5 INGREDIENT FREEZER BISCUITS

Prep Time: 10 mins
Cook Time: 22 mins
Total Time: 32 mins
Servings: 12

### *Ingredients*

- 2.5 cups all-purpose flour (plus some for dusting)
- 1 tsp salt
- 1 Tbsp sugar
- 4 tsp baking powder
- 1 pint heavy whipping cream

### *Instructions*

- In a large bowl, stir together the flour, salt, sugar, and baking powder until well combined.
- Pour in the heavy cream and stir until a sticky ball of dough forms. Sprinkle the dough generously with flour and then turn the dough out onto a floured surface. Gently knead the dough 2-3 times, or just until the dough feels mixed and has enough flour that it is no longer sticky. Avoid over working the dough.
- Gently pat the dough down into a 6x8 rectangle, then fold it in half. Repeat this two more times.

Folding the dough in this manner helps create layers within the biscuits.
- After folding, pat the dough down into a 6x8 rectangle one final time. The dough should be about one inch thick. Cut the dough into 12 squares.
- Line a baking sheet with parchment, then place the cut biscuits on the parchment, separated just slightly. Cover with plastic wrap and freeze the biscuits for a couple of hours, or just until solid. Label and date a gallon-sized freezer bag. Place the frozen biscuits in the bag for long term storage (3-4 months).
- To bake the biscuits, place any number of biscuits you want on a baking sheet lined with parchment. Let the biscuits thaw only as long as it takes to preheat the oven to 400ºF. Once the oven is preheated, bake the biscuits until puffed up tall and deep golden brown on top. Depending on your oven and size of the biscuits, it should take about 18-22 minutes (frozen), or 16-20 minutes (fresh).

### *Nutrition Info*

Calories: 255.52kcal, Carbohydrates: 20.16g, Protein: 2.5g, Fat: 16g, Sodium: 356.68mg, Fiber: 0.83g

# 94 ANNE BYRN'S 1917 APPLESAUCE CAKE

Prep Time: 15 mins
Cook Time: 35 mins
Total Time: 50 mins
Servings: 9, 1 piece each

## *Ingredients*

- 1 cup sugar
- 2 Tbsp butter (plus some for the pan)
- 1 cup unsweetened applesauce
- 2 cups all-purpose flour (plus 1 Tbsp)
- 1 tsp baking soda
- 1/2 tsp cinnamon
- 1/2 tsp ground cloves
- 1/4 tsp salt
- 1/4 tsp nutmeg
- 2/3 cup raisins

## *Instructions*

- Allow the butter to come to room temperature. Preheat the oven to 350ºF. Coat the inside of an 8x8-inch baking dish with butter.
- In a large bowl, cream together 2 Tbsp of butter and the sugar using a hand mixer or mixing by hand with a wooden spoon. Add the applesauce and stir to combine.

- In a separate bowl, stir together the flour, baking soda, cinnamon, cloves, salt, and nutmeg until well combined.
- Pour the flour mixture into the applesauce mixture and stir just until combined.
- In a separate small bowl, toss the raisins with about 1 Tbsp flour until they are lightly coated. Fold the flour coated raisins into the cake batter. Spread the cake batter into the prepared baking dish.
- Bake the cake for 30-35 minutes, or until the the center springs back when pressed. Let the cake cool for 15 minutes before slicing into 9 pieces.

**Nutrition Info**

Calories: 262.73kcal, Carbohydrates: 54.61g, Protein: 3.13g, Fat: 3.86g, Sodium: 240.04mg, Fiber: 2.17g

## 95 LEMON BUTTER GREEN BEANS

Prep Time: 10 mins
Cook Time: 7 mins
Total Time: 17 mins
Servings: 4

### *Ingredients*

- 1 lb. green beans
- 1 Tbsp butter
- 1 lemon
- Salt and Freshly Cracked Pepper to taste

### *Instructions*

- Use a microplane, zester, or small-holed cheese grater to remove the thin layer of yellow zest from the lemon. Set the zest aside. Remove the stems from the green beans and, if you prefer shorter pieces, snap them in half. Place the green beans in a colander and rinse well with cool water.
- Transfer the rinsed green beans to a deep skillet. Add about one inch of fresh water (the water will not cover the beans). Place a lid on the skillet and turn the flame on to medium-high. Allow the water to come up to a boil. Let the beans simmer and steam for 3-5 minutes, or just

until the beans are bright green and just slightly tender. Test the texture with a fork.
- Once the green beans are bright green and slightly tender, turn off the heat and drain them in a colander. Return the drained green beans to the still-warm skillet with the heat turned off.
- Add the butter, about 1/2 tsp of lemon zest, a quick squeeze of the lemon juice (about 1 tsp), a pinch of salt, and some freshly cracked pepper. Toss the green beans to distribute the seasonings and allow the residual heat to melt the butter.
- When the butter has melted fully, taste the green beans and add more salt, pepper, lemon juice, or lemon zest to your liking. Serve immediately.

### *Nutrition Info*

Calories: 150.2kcal, Carbohydrates: 22.1g, Protein: 4.43g, Fat: 5.98g, Sodium: 1270.45mg, Fiber: 6.73g

# 96 MANGO COCONUT TOFU BOWLS

Prep Time: 30 mins
Cook Time: 30 mins
Total Time: 1 hr
Servings: 4

## *Ingredients*

### SAVORY COCONUT RICE

- 1.5 cups uncooked jasmine or basmati rice
- 1 clove garlic, minced
- 3/4 tsp salt
- 1 13.5oz. can coconut milk
- 1 cup water

### HONEY LIME GLAZE

- 1 lime
- 1/4 cup honey
- 1/2 Tbsp soy sauce
- 1 tsp corn starch

### PAN FRIED TOFU

- 1 14oz. package firm or extra firm tofu
- 1 pinch salt
- 2 Tbsp corn starch

- 2 Tbsp neutral oil for frying

BOWL TOPPINGS

- 1 mango
- 1 avocado, sliced
- 2-3 green onions, sliced
- 1 pinch crushed red pepper
- 1 handful fresh cilantro

## *Instructions*

- Begin by pressing the tofu. Remove the tofu from the package, draining away all moisture. Wrap the tofu in a clean, lint-free dish towel or a few layers of paper towel. Place the wrapped tofu between two plates and place something heavy on top (cast iron pan or pot full of water). Let the tofu press for at least 30 minutes.
- To make the Savory Coconut Rice, combine the uncooked rice, minced garlic, salt, coconut milk, and water in a medium pot. Place a lid on the pot and bring to a boil over high heat. Once it reaches a boil, turn the heat down to low and let simmer for 20 minutes. Turn the heat off and let the pot sit, undisturbed, for 10 more minutes. Fluff the rice with a fork and set aside.
- While the rice is cooking, prepare the honey lime glaze. Use a zester, microplane, or small-holed

cheese grater to remove the thin layer of green zest from the lime. Squeeze the juice from the lime into a separate bowl (you'll need about 1/4 cup juice). Combine the juice with 1/2 tsp of the zest, honey, soy sauce, and corn starch in a bowl. Stir until the corn starch and honey are dissolved.
- After the tofu has been pressed, cut it into 1/2 inch cubes. Blot with a paper towel if needed to make sure the surface is dry. Season the tofu with a pinch of salt. Sprinkle the corn starch over top and gently toss until all the pieces are well coated.
- Heat the oil in a large skillet over medium heat until the oil is shimmering. Add the tofu and fry on until golden brown on each side (about 3 minutes each side). Remove the fried tofu from the pan and turn the heat down to low. While the tofu fries, cut the mango into cubes.
- Give the prepared glaze a quick stir, then add it to the skillet. Allow the glaze to begin to simmer, at which point it will thicken. Once thickened, turn the heat off and add the fried tofu and cubed mango. Toss to coat in the glaze.
- To build the bowls, place about one cup of the savory coconut rice in the bottom of each bowl, then top with a scoop of the mango and tofu. Add sliced green onions, sliced avocado, a pinch of red pepper flakes, and a few sprigs of cilantro on top of each bowl.

***Nutrition Info***

Calories: 655.73kcal, Carbohydrates: 101.45g, Protein: 17.25g, Fat: 21.85g, Sodium: 704.25mg, Fiber: 8.15g

## 97 MAPLE BROWN BUTTER MASHED SWEET POTATOES

Prep Time: 15 mins
Cook Time: 20 mins
Total Time: 35 mins
Servings: 6 cups

### *Ingredients*

- 3 lbs sweet potatoes
- 6 Tbsp butter*
- 1/4 cup real maple syrup
- 1/4 tsp cinnamon
- 1/8 tsp nutmeg
- 1/8 tsp ground cloves
- 1/4 cup chopped pecans

### *Instructions*

- Peel and dice the sweet potatoes. Add them to a large pot and cover with water. Place a lid on the pot and bring the water up to a boil over high heat. Boil the potatoes until they are very tender when pierced with a fork (5-10 minutes depending on the size of your sweet potato cubes). Drain the sweet potatoes and then mash until mostly smooth. Set the mashed sweet potatoes aside.

- Cut the butter into equal-sized pieces. Place the butter in a light colored skillet or pot. Place the skillet over medium-low heat and let it melt and being to foam. Continue to cook the butter, stirring constantly, until the butter solids begin to brown. Watch the butter closely once it begins to change color and remove it from the heat when it reaches a deep brown color and smells nutty or caramel-like. Immediately pour the butter into a separate bowl to stop the cooking process.
- Stir the maple syrup into the butter. Pour the maple syrup and butter mixture into the mashed sweet potatoes. Reserve 1-2 Tbsp of the maple brown butter to drizzle over top as a garnish. Also add the cinnamon, nutmeg, and cloves to the mashed potatoes, then stir to combine. Taste the sweet potatoes and adjust the syrup, spices, or salt if needed. Sprinkle the chopped pecans over top and drizzle the remaining maple brown butter just before serving.

### *Nutrition Info*

Calories: 362.73kcal, Carbohydrates: 55.22g, Protein: 4g, Fat: 14.5g, Sodium: 216.5mg, Fiber: 7.35g

# 98 SAVORY CABBAGE PANCAKES (OKONOMIYAKI)

Prep Time: 20 mins
Cook Time: 20 mins
Total Time: 40 mins
Servings: 6-inch pancakes

## Ingredients

PANCAKES

- 2 extra large eggs
- 1/2 cup water
- 1.5 Tbsp soy sauce
- 1 Tbsp toasted sesame oil
- 3/4 to 1 cup all-purpose flour
- 4-5 cups shredded green cabbage
- 1 carrot
- 3 green onions
- 2 Tbsp oil for frying

TOPPINGS

- 1/4 cup mayonnaise
- 2 Tbsp sriracha
- 1/2 Tbsp sesame seeds
- 2 green onions

*Instructions*

- Remove any wilted leaves from the outside of the cabbage. Cut the cabbage into quarters and remove the core. Thinly slice or shred half of the cabbage, or until you have 4-5 cups shredded cabbage. Peel the carrot and shred it using a large-holed cheese grater. Slice the green onions.
- In a large bowl, whisk together the eggs, water, soy sauce, and sesame oil until smooth. Begin whisking in the flour, 1/4 cup at a time, until it forms a thick, smooth batter (about 3/4 to 1 cup total flour).
- Add the cabbage, carrots, and green onion to the batter and stir until the vegetables are mixed and everything is evenly coated in batter.
- Heat 1/2 Tbsp oil in a non-stick or cast iron skillet over medium heat. Once hot, add 3/4 cup of the vegetable and batter mixture. Press it down into the hot skillet to form a circle, about 6 inches in diameter and 1/2 inch thick. Place a cover on the skillet to hold in the steam, which will help the cabbage soften as it cooks. Cook the pancake until golden brown on the bottom (3-5 minutes), then flip and cook until golden brown on the second side. Pile the cooked pancakes on a plate and cover with foil to keep warm until ready to eat. Add more oil to the skillet as needed as you cook the pancakes.

- To prepare the sriracha mayo, mix together 1/4 cup mayonnaise and 2 Tbsp sriracha in a small bowl. Drizzle the sriracha mayo over the pancakes just before serving, followed with a sprinkle of sesame seeds and sliced green onion.

***Nutrition Info***

Calories: 263.32kcal, Carbohydrates: 23.6g, Protein: 5.9g, Fat: 16.65g, Sodium: 449.58mg, Fiber: 2.95g

## 99 PASTA WITH 5 INGREDIENT BUTTER TOMATO SAUCE

Prep Time: 5 mins
Cook Time: 45 mins
Total Time: 50 mins
Servings: 4

### Ingredients

TOASTED BREAD CRUMBS (optional)

- 2 Tbsp olive oil
- 1/2 cup breadcrumbs
- 1/4 tsp salt
- 1/2 tsp dried oregano
- Freshly cracked Pepper

PASTA WITH BUTTER TOMATO SAUCE

- 8 oz. pasta
- 4 Tbsp salted butter
- 3 cloves garlic
- 28 oz. can whole peeled tomatoes
- 1/2 tsp salt (or to taste)
- Freshly cracked pepper

### Instructions

- To make the toasted bread crumbs, heat the olive oil in a large skillet over medium heat. Once the oil is shimmering, add the bread crumbs, salt, oregano, and some freshly cracked pepper. Cook and stir the bread crumbs continuously until they achieve a deep golden color. Remove them from the skillet and let cool until ready to use.
- To make the sauce, mince the garlic and add it to a large deep skillet with the butter. Sauté the garlic in the butter over medium heat for about a minute, or just until it becomes fragrant. Add the can of tomatoes, along with all the juices, and some freshly cracked pepper. Break the tomatoes up into a few chunks with your spoon (they should be soft and easily crushed).
- Stir the ingredients in the skillet, then let it come up to a simmer. Once it reaches a simmer, reduce the heat to medium-low and let it continue to simmer, without a lid, for about 30 minutes. Stir the sauce occasionally as it simmers, breaking the tomatoes into smaller pieces as you stir.
- While the sauce simmers, cook the pasta according to the package directions. Save about 1/2 cup of the starchy cooking water before draining the pasta in a colander.
- After simmering for 30 minutes, the sauce should have thickened and become slightly less

acidic and slightly more sweet. Season the sauce with a final 1/2 tsp of salt (or to your liking). Add the cooked and drained pasta to the sauce and toss to coat. Use some of the reserved starchy cooking water to loosen the pasta if it becomes too dry. Top the pasta and sauce with a generous sprinkle of toasted bread crumbs, then serve.

**Nutrition Info**

Calories: 468.2kcal, Carbohydrates: 61.73g, Protein: 10.88g, Fat: 19.13g, Sodium: 1023.58mg, Fiber: 4.08g

# 100 LEMON BERRY COBBLER

Prep Time: 15 mins
Cook Time: 25 mins
Total Time: 40 mins
Servings: 4

## Ingredients

BERRY LAYER

- 12 oz. frozen mixed berries, thawed
- 1/4 cup sugar
- 1 1/2 Tbsp cornstarch
- 1 fresh lemon

BISCUIT TOPPING

- 1 cup all-purpose flour
- 1 tsp baking powder
- 1/4 cup sugar
- 1/8 tsp salt
- 4 Tbsp cold butter
- 5 Tbsp milk*

## Instructions

- Preheat the oven to 425ºF. Use a zester, microplane, or small-holed cheese grater to remove the zest from the lemon.
- Place the thawed berries in a bowl and add the sugar, cornstarch, about 1/2 tsp of the zest, and 1 Tbsp of the lemon juice. Stir to combine. Pour the prepared berries and all the juices into a small casserole dish (4 cup capacity).
- In a medium bowl, stir together the flour, baking powder, sugar, salt, and another 1/2 tsp of the lemon zest. Cut the butter into small pieces, then add it to the flour mixture. Use your hands to work the butter into the flour until the butter is in very small pieces and the mixture resembles damp sand. Add the milk and stir until a slightly sticky dough forms.
- Drop the biscuit dough onto the berries in small pieces. It's okay if the dough does not completely cover the berries.
- Bake the cobbler in the preheated oven for 20-25 minutes, or until the top is golden brown and the berries are bubbling up around the edges. To prevent messes from the berry juices bubbling over, place the casserole dish on a baking sheet covered with parchment to catch any spills.
- Serve warm topped with ice cream or whipped cream, if desired. Garnish with any remaining lemon zest.

***Nutrition Info***

Calories: 378.45kcal, Carbohydrates: 63.33g, Protein: 4.53g, Fat: 13.1g, Sodium: 358.18mg, Fiber: 3.78g

# 101 ZUCCHINI AND ORZO SALAD WITH CHIMICHURRI

Prep Time: 20 mins
Cook Time: 15 mins
Total Time: 35 mins
Servings: 4

## *Ingredients*

CHIMICHURRI

- 1/2 cup olive oil
- 1/4 cup red wine vinegar
- 1 cup Italian (flat leaf) parsley, packed
- 1/2 cup cilantro*, packed
- 3 cloves garlic
- 1 tsp dried oregano
- 1/2 tsp cumin
- 1/4 tsp red pepper flakes
- 1/2 tsp salt

SALAD

- 1 cup uncooked orzo
- 1 medium zucchini (0.75 to 1 lb.)
- Pinch of salt and pepper
- 1 pint grape or cherry tomatoes

## Instructions

- Prepare the chimichurri by washing the parsley and cilantro leaves well, then shaking off as much water as possible. Pull the leaves from the stems and add them to a food processor, along with the olive oil, vinegar, garlic, oregano, cumin, red pepper, and salt. Pulse the mixture until smooth. (Or finely mince the parsley, cilantro, and garlic with a knife and stir together with the remaining ingredients.)
- Cook the orzo according to the package directions, drain in a colander, and then let cool.
- Slice the zucchini into 1/4 inch thick rounds. The zucchini can be added to the salad raw, grilled, or roasted in the oven first. I used a countertop grill to grill the slices, then cut them into quarter rounds after grilling. If roasting in the oven, toss with a little oil, a pinch of salt and pepper, then roast at 400 degrees for about 20 minutes. Let the zucchini cool slightly.
- While the zucchini and pasta are cooling, slice the grape tomatoes in half. Once the zucchini and orzo are no longer steaming hot, combine them in a bowl with the tomatoes. Pour about half of the chimichurri over top, and then toss until everything is coated. Add more chimichurri to your liking (I used about 3/4 of the batch). Taste and add salt or pepper to the salad if needed.

# CONCLUSION

All people who suffer from fibromyalgia are overwhelmed by its variety of symptoms. Fibromyalgia is considered to be a serious neurological condition that in time can lead to many complications. Although millions of people worldwide are confronted with fibromyalgia, the exact causes of the disorder haven't yet been clarified. Despite the fact that scientists have been able to establish a connection between abnormal brain activity and the symptoms of fibromyalgia, the factors responsible for causing the disorder are still unknown.

The factors of risk that are considered to facilitate the occurrence and the development of fibromyalgia are stress, depression, inadequate sleeping patterns, inappropriate diet and unhealthy lifestyle. Although many people who are exposed to all of these factors of risk don't develop neurological conditions, statistics indicate that all patients diagnosed with fibromyalgia have suffered from depression at certain stages of their lives and many of them have developed the disorder on the premises of insomnia, unhealthy lifestyle and inappropriate diet.

An appropriate diet is vital for maintaining both physical and mental balance and it can strengthen the immune system of the organism. A good fibromyalgia diet can be a very effective way of overcoming the symptoms of the disorder, normalizing and stimulating the activity of the body. Unhealthy lifestyle, stress, lack of sleep, smoking, the abuse of alcoholic beverages are all considered to be factors of risk in the development of fibromyalgia. By improving your lifestyle and by respecting an appropriate fibromyalgia diet, you will quickly feel improvements in your health. Also, an effective fibromyalgia diet can considerably ameliorate the symptoms of the disorder. Here are some tips in establishing an effective fibromyalgia diet:

- A good fibromyalgia diet should exclude alcoholic beverages and smoking; also, caffeine is known to have undesirable effects on the fragile nervous system of people with fibromyalgia and therefore, all products containing caffeine (coffee, tea, carbonated soda, cocoa and chocolate) should be excluded from the fibromyalgia diet.
- An appropriate fibromyalgia diet should contain less dairy products, especially those that contain high levels of fat; consider using soy replacements instead (soy milk, tofu).
- Consume less wheat products, as they are not well tolerated by people with fibromyalgia.
- Reduce the amount of sugar in your fibromyalgia diet.

- Stay away from food products that contain additives, colorants and preservatives.
- Avoid any kind of fried foods; consider eating more boiled and baked foods instead.
- Add more home-made meals in your fibromyalgia diet; consume more soups, as they are better tolerated by the stomach.
- Consume more liquids.
- Reduce the amount of salt and spices in your meals.
- Reduce the amount of meat in your fibromyalgia diet.
- Consume plenty of vegetables and fruits, as they are a vital source of vitamins and minerals.
- Consider taking mineral and vitamin supplements.

These are some basic tips in establishing a good, effective fibromyalgia diet. By respecting these suggestions in planning your fibromyalgia diet, you will soon begin to feel an amelioration of your symptoms. A good fibromyalgia diet can correct the sleeping problems that occur to most people with the disorder, also diminishing fatigue and the lack of energy characteristic to fibromyalgia.

Printed in Great Britain
by Amazon